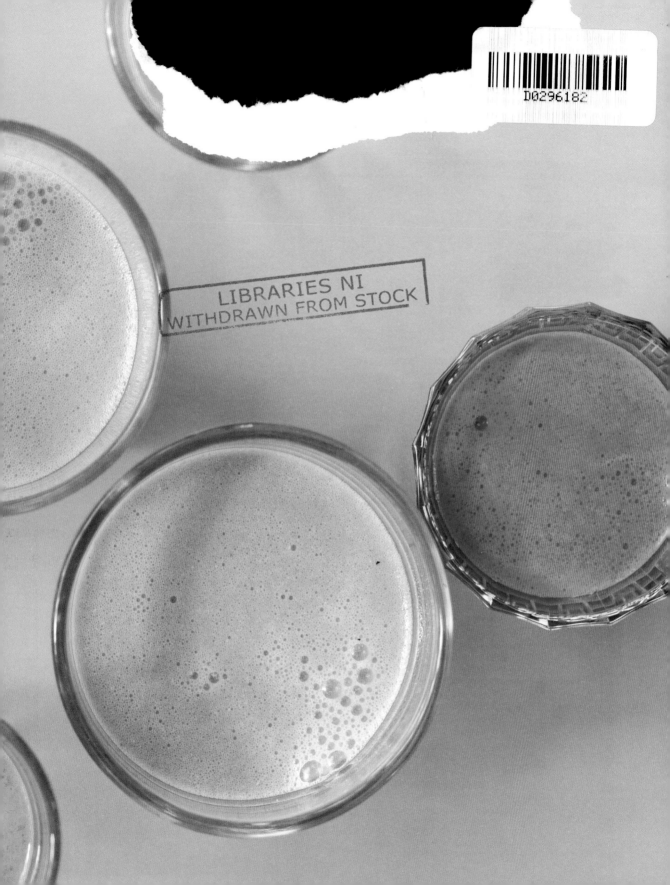

SUPERFOOD
Juices and Smoothies

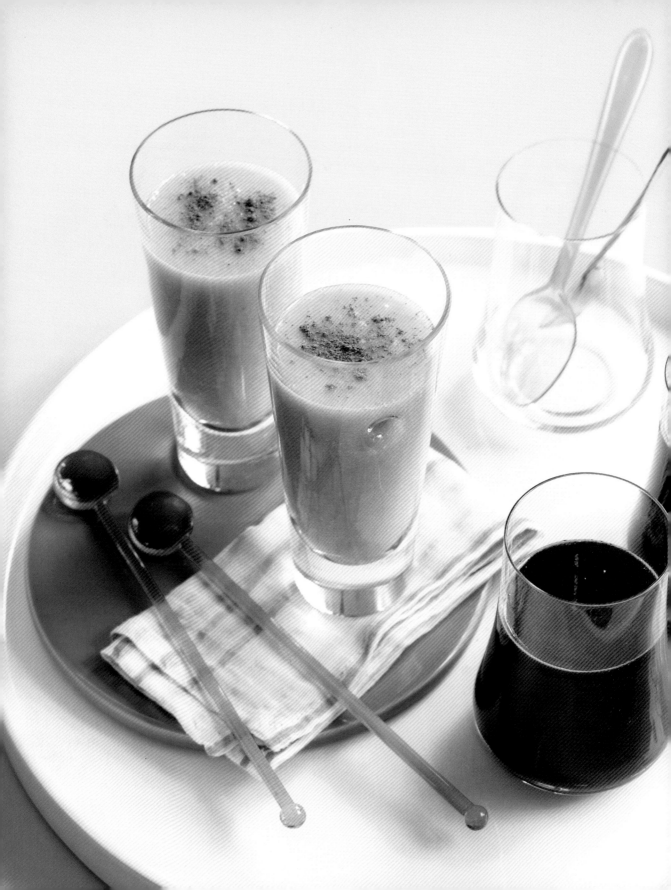

SUPERFOOD
Juices and Smoothies

Over 100 recipes for all-natural
fruit and vegetable drinks
with added super nutrients

Nicola Graimes

photography by
Kate Whitaker

RYLAND PETERS & SMALL
LONDON • NEW YORK

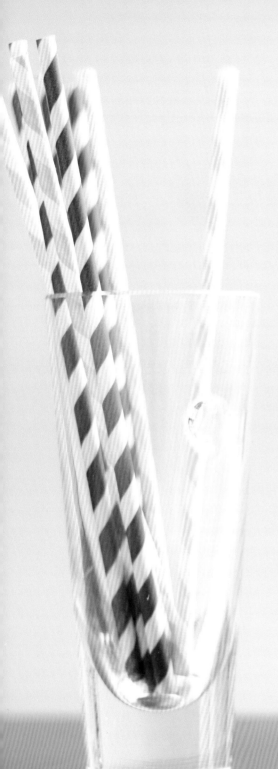

Editor Miriam Catley
Senior Designers Toni Kay
 and Megan Smith
Head of Production
 Patricia Harrington
Art Director Leslie Harrington
Editorial Director Julia Charles

Food Stylist Lucy McKelvie
Props Stylist Liz Belton
Indexer Hilary Bird

First published in 2014.
This edition published in 2018
by Ryland Peters & Small
20–21 Jockey's Fields
London WC1R 4BW
and
Ryland Peters & Small, Inc.
341 E 116th St, New York NY 10029
www.rylandpeters.com

10 9 8 7 6 5 4 3 2 1

Text © Nicola Graimes 2014, 2018
Design and photographs
© Ryland Peters & Small 2014,
2018

ISBN: 978 1 84975 931 1

Printed and bound in China

A CIP record for this book is
available from the British Library.

US Library of Congress cataloging-
in-publication data has been
applied for.

Neither the author nor the
publisher can be held responsible
for any claim arising out of the
information in this book. Always
consult your health advisor or
doctor if you have any concerns
about your health or nutrition.

Notes
• The recipes have been created
with adults in mind; if serving them
to children omit the superfoods
and dilute half and half with pure
or filtered water.
• All spoon measurements are
level, unless otherwise specified.
• When a recipe calls for frozen
fruit there is no need to defrost
the fruit before using.

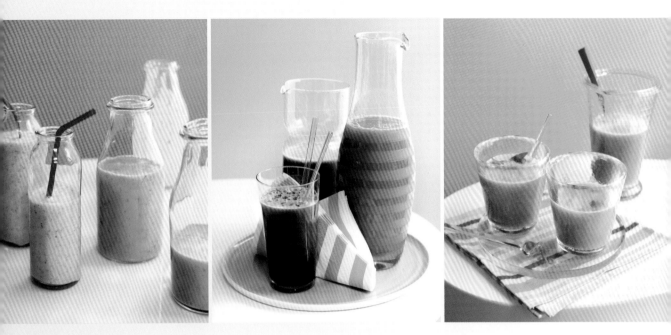

Contents

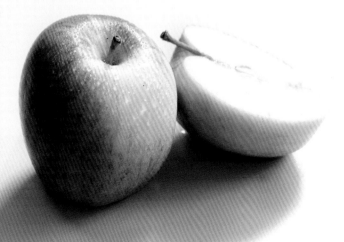

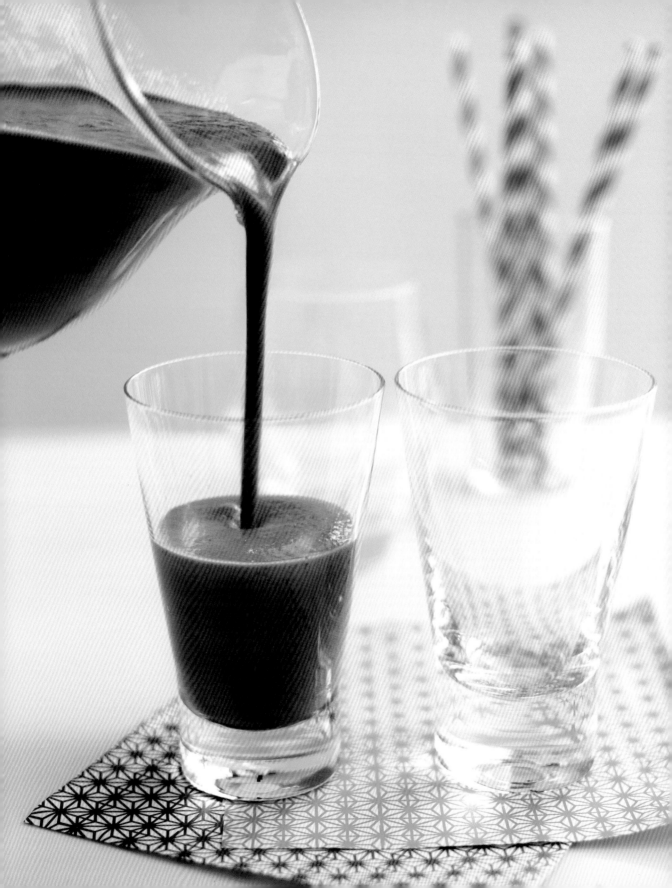

Introduction

By enjoying fresh, raw juices, smoothies and blends on a regular basis you are on the path to good health and with the addition of superfoods you are on the superhighway to rejuvenating and invigorating both mind and body. Whether you're looking for a potent pick-me-up, an effective detoxifier or an anti-ageing rejuvenator, this book shows how to make flavour-packed juices, smoothies and blends with these – and many other – therapeutic properties. But what makes this juicing book different from so many others is that, along with the nutrients gleaned from fresh fruit and vegetables, these great-tasting drinks contain the added benefit of active superfoods, or super-nutrients, such as spirulina, wheatgrass, maca, baobab, açaí berries, chia seeds and cacao nibs among others. To help those unfamiliar with these superfoods there is an in-depth list with a detailed explanation of their numerous health benefits.

Alongside over 100 recipes this book gives invaluable, practical advice plus tips on how to choose and what to look for when buying a juicer or blender to best suit your needs. There are also hints for getting the most from your fresh produce, including shopping advice, as well as storing and preparation. For those who want to start from scratch, there are recipes for making-your-own natural yogurt and nut milk as well as information on how to sprout seeds and beans so you can rest assured that your fantastic juice or smoothie is not only nutritious but also 100 per cent home-produced.

There is no comparison between home-produced juices and shop-bought from a health point of view; with homemade drinks you know what you're getting, you can choose your favourite fresh produce, they are additive-free with no added sugar and they're not pasteurised, which can deplete their nutritional status. Homemade juices can be described as liquid fuel, nourishing the body with a potent combination of vitamins, minerals, antioxidants, phytochemicals and enzymes. As well as giving a nutritional boost, juices, smoothies and blends have the ability to cleanse the liver and kidneys, revitalise flagging energy levels, flush the body of toxins, boost immunity, de-stress, rejuvenate the mind and body and aid weight-loss. These nutritional properties are flagged in each recipe alongside an explanation of key health benefits and nutrients. The recipes are divided into the following chapters: Detoxifiers; Energy-enhancers; Pick-me-ups; Weight-loss Aids; and Beauty Boosters. For easy-reference, each chapter is split into refreshing juices, soothing smoothies and rejuvenating blends, with each one featuring an added active ingredient. And, perhaps most importantly, they all taste great.

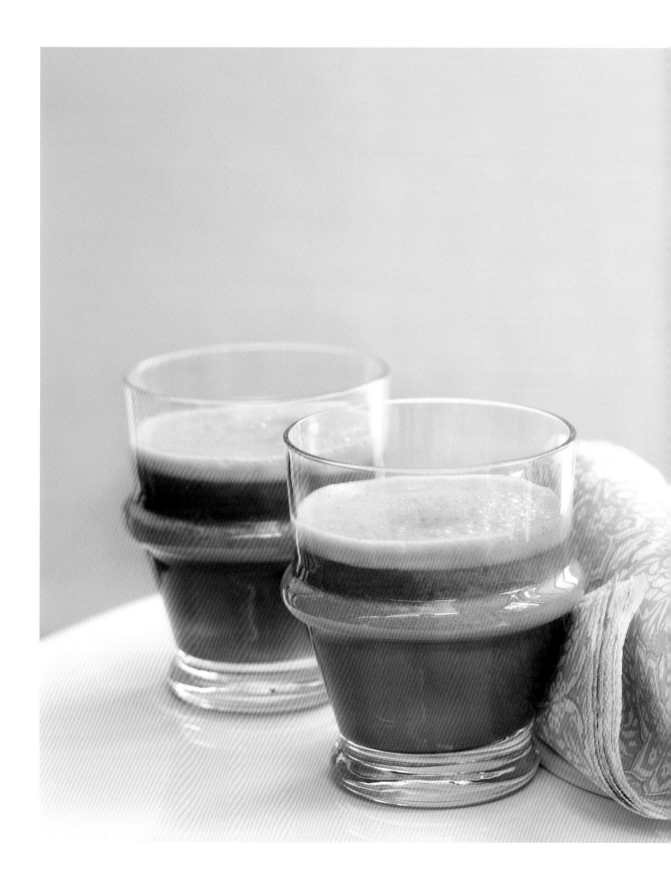

The juice kitchen

Juicing basics

To ensure that you get the most from your juicer or blender, let's go back to basics by explaining the difference between a juice, smoothie and blend. The former is made by passing fresh raw vegetables or fruit through a juicer, which extracts the fibre to provide a readily digestible, nutrient-laden juice. Smoothies, on the other hand, are made by pulverising fresh raw produce into a pulp in a blender with yogurt, milk or a dairy-free alternative, while a blended drink replaces the dairy element with juice, water and the like; either way the end result is thicker than a juice and also retains valuable fibre, although the nutrients take longer for the body to absorb.

• Choose fresh produce that is in season and at the peak of ripeness as the juice, smoothie or blend will not only taste superior but will also be at its nutritional best. Conversely, avoid under-ripe, old, wrinkly or damaged fruit and vegetables. It's advisable to buy fresh produce from a retailer with a steady turnover. Better still, grow or pick-your-own!

• One of the goals of drinking juices is to flush out toxins from the body so it makes sense to avoid using foods that contain unwanted additives, chemicals, pesticides and fertilizers and use organic fresh produce instead. If the purse allows, the health benefits and often the taste are well worth the extra cost. If using non-organic fresh produce, wash it well. Also choose unwaxed citrus fruit or alternatively scrub it thoroughly before use.

• It's not always necessary to remove the skin from fresh produce before blending and as most of the nutrients lie in, or just below, the skin it pays to leave it on whenever possible (obviously if the skin is very thick or inedible this isn't an option). The skin will make the blend slightly fibrous, but I don't usually find this an issue when you take into account the health benefits.

• Some juicers may struggle with leafy vegetables and herbs, so an easy solution is to roll them into a bundle or wrap them around a more juicy vegetable or fruit before putting them through the machine. For maximum juice extraction if you have a centrifugal juicer (see page 12), soft or particularly juicy fruit and vegetables, such as berries, peaches, pears, melon or cucumber, can be put through the appliance twice.

• Juices, smoothies and blends don't tend to keep well and should be drunk soon after making as their flavour, texture and nutritional value diminish with exposure to light and oxygen. You can add lemon juice to extend their life slightly, but I find they are still best consumed shortly after making.

• Fresh juices can be strong-tasting and potent, so if you have a delicate digestive system or are not used to drinking them, dilute with pure or filtered water before drinking. The recipes have been created with adults in mind; if serving them to children omit the superfoods and dilute half and half with pure or filtered water.

• Superfoods can be bought in various forms from fresh to tablets, capsules and powders. For convenience and consistency, the recipes in this book use them in powdered form. The dosage given in each recipe is perhaps conservative, but if you haven't taken superfoods before it's advisable to start off small and then increase the dosage after a period of time when your body becomes more attuned and after monitoring any reaction. It's also recommended to compare the quantity of superfood specified in the recipe with the dosage on the pack as strengths can vary. For herbal remedies, again check the recommended dosage on the pack.

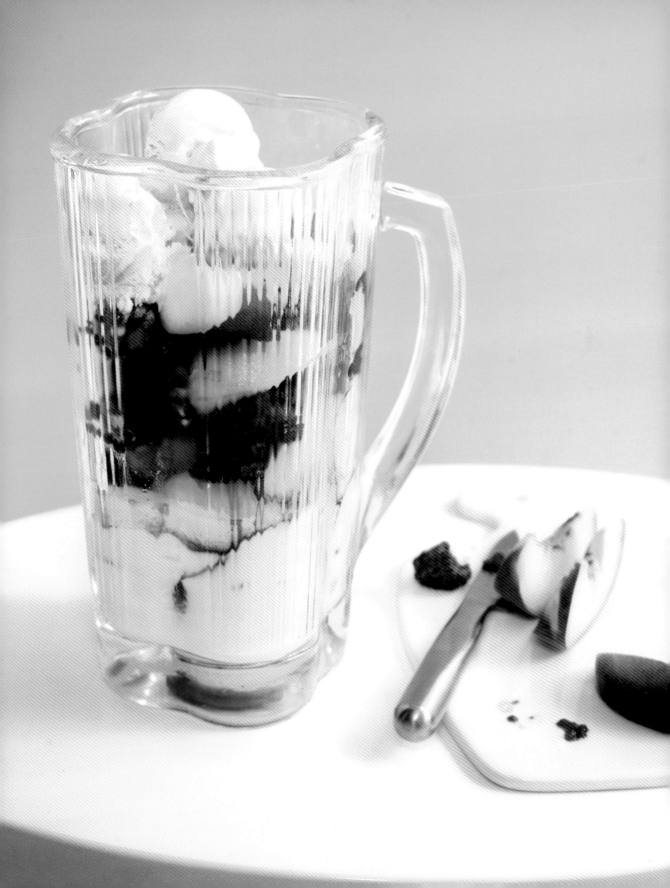

Equipment and tools

Juicers and blenders have come a long way in recent years but which piece of equipment you choose to buy largely depends on your budget and what you need from your appliance.

Centrifugal juicer

This juicer works by using a flat cutting blade in the bottom of a rapidly spinning basket, which shreds the fresh produce and flings the pulp to the sides of the basket, or in a separate container, while the juice passes through the small holes into a jug/jar. If you are making a small amount of juice, there is an advantage to using a centrifugal machine as it doesn't eject the pulp but continues to work until the basket is full, so it reduces the amount of cleaning. This type of appliance does vary in its juice yields, but it is a quick and convenient way of juicing. Choose

a model with a robust, high-powered motor to handle the high-speed extraction process.

Masticating juicer

This type of juicer effectively shreds or 'chews' vegetables and fruit, releasing their juice and the nutrients that go with it. It is extremely effective in extracting juice and tends to be more proficient at handling leafy greens and herbs than a centrifugal model. However, for some people, it is preferable to have a juicer and a separate wheatgrass/leafy greens machine, possibly hand-operated, to cover all bases. Masticating juicers tend to produce juices with a reasonable nutritional shelf life as they incorporate less oxygen in the juicing process than centrifugal machines. Opt for a sturdy appliance with a reliable, powerful motor and it should last

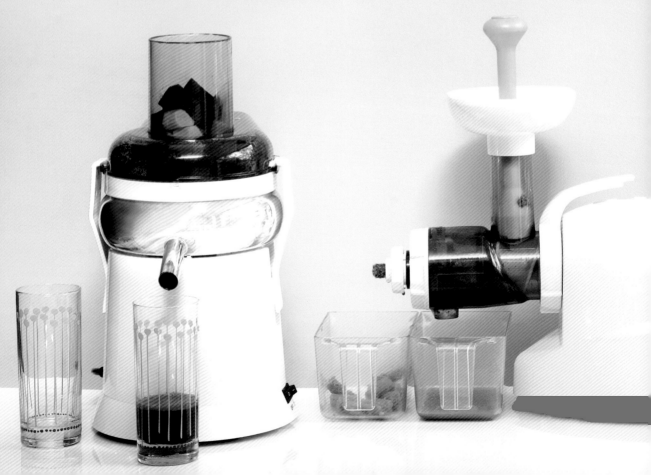

you for many years. Also choose one that is easy to clean and put back together afterwards. Most machines come with various attachments that allow you to make ice cream, mill grains and grind nuts, for instance, so it's worth bearing this in mind when considering your options.

Blender

If you intend to use your blender on a regular basis it pays to invest in a sturdy, heavy-based model with a powerful motor as it will certainly make light work of smoothies and blended drinks that include firm fruit and vegetables. Other factors you may wish to consider are whether the jug/jar is the right capacity for your needs and that it is sturdy with a tight-fitting lid and a hole in the top for adding ingredients. It should also be easy to clean. You may not need a plethora of speeds but look for an appliance with a range of functions, 3 or 4 speeds and a pulse button; many blenders also have pre-programmed cycles that make them easy and convenient to use, as well as attachments that can grind nuts and spices or mill grains.

Citrus juicer

Expensive equipment is not essential for making citrus juices. The hand-held reamer, citrus squeezer or the more costly citrus press are perfect for extracting juice from oranges, lemons and limes. Many electrical juicers also come with an attachment that can extract the juice from citrus fruit.

Hand-held blender

A hand-held immersion blender is perfect for handling an individual serving of a smoothie or blend as well as pulverising herbs or greens to stir into juices if your juicer has difficulty coping with fresh leafy stuff. As with a blender, look for a sturdy appliance offering variable speeds and one that is easy to clean.

chlorella

hemp protein powder

wheatgrass

Superfoods

Superfoods (or super-nutrients) are the buzz-word of the moment. This collection of potent, nutrient-rich, bioavailable foods is believed to be essential for optimal health, both of body and mind. If taken regularly, they help to correct imbalances in the body, strengthening immunity and cleansing and rejuvenating the system. The following list details the superfoods used in the recipes in this book in alphabetical order for easy reference. It isn't exhaustive as 'new' superfoods regularly come to our attention, but this makes them all the more exciting.

Açaí berry

A purple, blueberry-looking fruit from the Amazon rainforest, the açaí berry is believed to aid weight-loss. It works by improving digestion, reducing cravings and boosting metabolism, enabling the body to process food more efficiently and consequently burn fat. The berries are also high in anti-ageing and energy-boosting antioxidants. Look for a good-quality, reputable brand. In a powdered form, açaí berries add both colour and a rich, slightly chocolaty flavour to smoothies, blends and juices.

Aloe vera

The leaves of this succulent plant contain a colourless, jelly-like substance that is trusted as

a topical treatment for burns, bites and abrasions, but if taken internally it supports the health of the digestive system, hydrates the skin and supports the immune system; quality is key when buying this vitamin- and mineral-rich supplement.

Baobab

Packed with vitamin C (around three times as much as found in an orange), this nutrient-dense African fruit boosts energy levels and the immune system as well as the health of the skin. It is also a good source of antioxidants, calcium, potassium and B vitamins. With its slightly sharp citrus flavour, baobab adds zing to vegetable- and fruit-based juices and tastes great in blended drinks.

Barleygrass

With similar therapeutic attributes as wheatgrass and brimming with vitamins and minerals (see page 18), barleygrass is slightly easier to digest and has a milder flavour than its cereal counterpart. This high-chlorophyll food acts as a free-radical scavenger and also reduces inflammation in the body. The recipes in this book use powdered barleygrass, but do use fresh, if available, and your juicer can cope with it, as its nutrient content is likely to be superior.

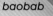

cranberry

purple corn

baobab

camu camu

Bee pollen

The tiny, golden nuggets of bee pollen are considered one of nature's most nourishing foods, being rich in protein, carbohydrate, vitamins and minerals. With its intense honey taste, bee pollen adds flavour to juices, smoothies and blends as well as texture when sprinkled over the top. It has an impressive list of therapeutic properties: boosting energy levels; supporting the immune system; as well as aiding digestion, respiration, the heart and circulation. It has also been used in the treatment of infertility problems and performs as an aphrodisiac.

Cacao (raw)

Raw cacao powder and nibs are very high in antioxidant flavonoids, magnesium, iron, zinc and essential fatty acids, which all promote good health and may reduce the risk of health problems as wide ranging as arthritis, cancer and heart disease. The theobromine found naturally in raw cacao is a mild stimulant, which lifts the mood and even curbs depression. It adds a rich, dark chocolate intensity to smoothies and blends.

Camu camu

The fruit from this South American plant is rich in vitamin C and other antioxidants and has been shown to possess impressive anti-inflammatory properties as well as an ability to boost the immune system. It's early days, but initial research shows that camu camu may help in the treatment of diabetes, fatigue, cancer, atherosclerosis and liver disease. It has a slightly caramel flavour.

Chia seeds

For its size, the tiny black chia seed packs a powerful punch: not only is it said to be the one of the richest plant sources of omega-3 fats, it is also a source of complete protein, containing all essential amino acids, fibre, antioxidants, vitamins and minerals. A staple food of the ancient Mayans and Aztecs, some nutritionists recommend soaking the seeds in a little water before use to increase bioavailability, but others say they are small enough to break down in the body.

Chlorella

This nutrient-rich green algae helps to detoxify, cleanse, alkalise and protect the body, boosting energy levels as well as vitality. Chlorella encourages cellular renewal, growth and repair, which all decline with age. It features the highest level of chlorophyll of any food, helping to control viral and fungal infections such as candida overgrowth, chronic fatigue and poor immunity. It is also an anti-inflammatory, relieving

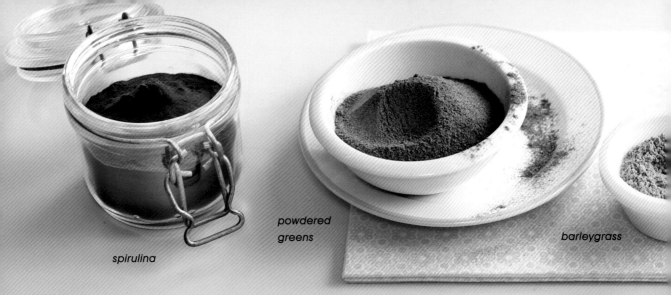

spirulina

powdered
greens

barleygrass

arthritis pain. Stress, depression, constipation, asthma, poor digestion and high blood pressure have all been found to improve after taking chlorella on a regular basis.

Chlorella contains a higher percentage of protein and beneficial fatty acids, including omega-3, than both wheatgrass and spirulina.

Detox greens powder/detox mix
(see Powdered greens)

Flaxseeds
Available as brown or golden seeds as well as ground into a coarse powder, flaxseeds are a beneficial plant source of omega-3 fatty acids. They are also an excellent source of the phytonutrient lignans and provide significant amounts of fibre, which benefits digestive health. Their antioxidant content has been linked to a reduced risk of heart disease as well as cancer of the breast, prostate and colon.

Goji berries
Known as the 'longevity fruit', goji berries may promote the production of human growth hormone (HGH), which influences the level of all hormones in the body. They are also a rich source of l-glutamine and l-arginine, two amino acids that work in tandem to rejuvenate the skin and boost the metabolism. That's not all, the red

berries act as a sexual tonic and are rich in lutein, which benefits the eyes and is essential for healthy vision. Goji help to alkalise the body, calming the nerves and negating stress.

Lacuma
This sub-tropical fruit makes a good sugar alternative as it's naturally sweet with a slight caramel flavour. It also provides a high concentration of antioxidants, calcium, iron, vitamins C and B3 and fibre as well as containing anti-inflammatory properties.

Maca
This root is native to South America and has been used for generations to boost energy levels, strength, fertility, balance hormones and enhance libido. Its ability to regulate hormone irregularities means it's particularly good for menopausal symptoms and menstruation. Maca has a pleasing malty taste and works well in creamy smoothies combined with yogurt or nut milk.

Manuka honey
This amazing, rich-tasting honey made from the flowers of the manuka bush, a native of New Zealand, possesses a range of healing properties that are over and above that of regular honey. Manuka has impressive anti-inflammatory, antibacterial and antifungal qualities, tackling

reishi

MSM
Methylsulfonylmethane

maca

even antibiotic-resistant bacterial strains such as MRSA. It is not fully understood why but not all manuka honey has the same potency, so it's important to buy a brand that is tested and verified with a UMF (Unique Manuka Factor) strength rating of level 10 and above, which indicates how active it is.

MSM (Methylsulfonylmethane)

This sulphur compound, found naturally in fruit, vegetables, dairy, meat and seafood, has been shown to improve the condition of the skin, hair and nails as well as strengthening collagen in the joints, thereby increasing flexibility. Initial studies show it may also help in the treatment of arthritis and inflammatory conditions.

Powdered greens

There are many different brands available and it pays to buy powdered greens from a reputable retailer and avoid those that include unwanted additives. They shouldn't be seen as a substitute for real leafy greens, but they are a great way of boosting your dietary intake and the nutritional value of juices, smoothies and blends. What's more, many blends contain other potent health ingredients such as chlorella, spirulina, wheatgrass, flaxseeds, alfalfa and probiotics so you get a super-nutritious conglomeration in one pot. The health benefits vary depending on what you want from your greens mix, so it's possible to buy blends for detoxing, energy-boosting, immunity support or improving digestion, for example.

Purple corn

Richer in antioxidants than blueberries, this Peruvian superfood has been shown to be brimming with phytonutrients as well as anthocyanins which promote collagen formation, improving the condition of the skin, hair, nails and joints. Anthocyanins encourage connective tissue regeneration as well as helping to stabilize and protect blood vessels from free radical damage. Furthermore, purple corn may protect against heart disease and reduce high blood pressure.

Reishi

In Chinese medicine, this prized fungus is known as the 'mushroom of immortality' for its wide-reaching, impressive list of therapeutic qualities. Its significant, immune-boosting properties have been shown to help prevent and treat cancer, heart disease and strokes, and also may have implications for treating those with AIDS and other immune system disorders. What's more, reishi can calm the nerves, aid sleep, rejuvenate the brain and maintain balance in the body. In its dried, powdered form, reishi has a rich, earthy mushroomy taste that works in more savoury juices, smoothies and blends.

Spirulina

This impressive, highly nutritious, nourishing blue-green micro algae both regenerates and cleanses the body. This is thanks to its rich chlorophyll content, which helps transport oxygen to every cell in the body. It is one of the highest sources of usable protein and features essential fatty acids, antioxidants, vitamins A, B12, E and K, iron, calcium and phytonutrients in a readily usable and digestible form. Spirulina has been found to treat liver damage, protect the kidneys, enrich the blood, protect the heart, enhance intestinal flora, aid weight loss and inhibit the growth of yeast, fungi and bacteria in the body; an all-round winning combination!

Wheatgrass

Widely acknowledged as one of nature's superfoods, wheatgrass contains high concentrations of vitamins, minerals, chlorophyll and all essential amino acids, along with digestive enzymes, some of which are not found in other foods. It is a well-known detoxifier, blood purifier and cleanser, but is perhaps less known for its cholesterol-reducing, anti-ageing and anti-inflammatory properties. The recipes in this book use wheatgrass powder, but you can buy wheatgrass in seed form to grow-your-own as well as pre-grown. Interestingly, wheatgrass is classified as a leafy green, rather than a grain, so it's suitable for those with wheat allergies.

Others...

Coconut water (and coconut milk drink)

This clear liquid found inside a young coconut has seen a huge growth in popularity, particularly as a low-sugar alternative to high-sugar energy sports drinks. Its high potassium, and electrolyte mineral content, prevents muscle cramps and spasms and effectively rehydrates the body. Most potent is the juice from a freshly opened coconut. The packaged version is a worthy alternative, but avoid those with added sugar. Coconut milk drink makes a creamy alternative to dairy milk

and is full of beneficial medium-chain fatty acids, said to be good for the heart, digestion, skin, hair and wellbeing.

Echinacea

If taken on a regular basis, this popular herbal remedy can stimulate the immune system and shorten the recovery time from colds and viruses.

Fruit powders

Fruit powders are made from pure fruit that has been freeze-dried. They make a convenient and healthy way to colour and flavour drinks. Generally a good source of vitamin C, cranberry in particular can help treat urinary tract infections.

Protein powders

Protein plays an essential role in the repair and maintenance of every cell in the body. We're not talking body-building whey powder here but plant-based proteins, such as those made from soya, hemp and pea. Stress, illness, hormonal imbalances and high activity all affect protein requirements, but it's also possible to eat too much so if your diet contains good amounts of protein, you may feel it unnecessary to supplement.

Milk thistle

The black seeds harvested from the milk thistle flower contain the active ingredient silymarin, which is effective in detoxifying the liver as well as protecting it against the damaging effects of toxins, alcohol and other elements. It promotes the regeneration and repair of liver cells and has been shown to reverse liver damage.

Probiotics

These beneficial bacteria improve the intestinal flora of the gut by inhibiting the growth of harmful bacteria. They are beneficial after a bout of food poisoning, a stomach bug or antibiotics. Research has shown that probiotics may also be able to treat diabetes, improve immunity and aid weight loss. Buy the best quality containing both *lactobacillus acidophilus* and *bifodobacterium*.

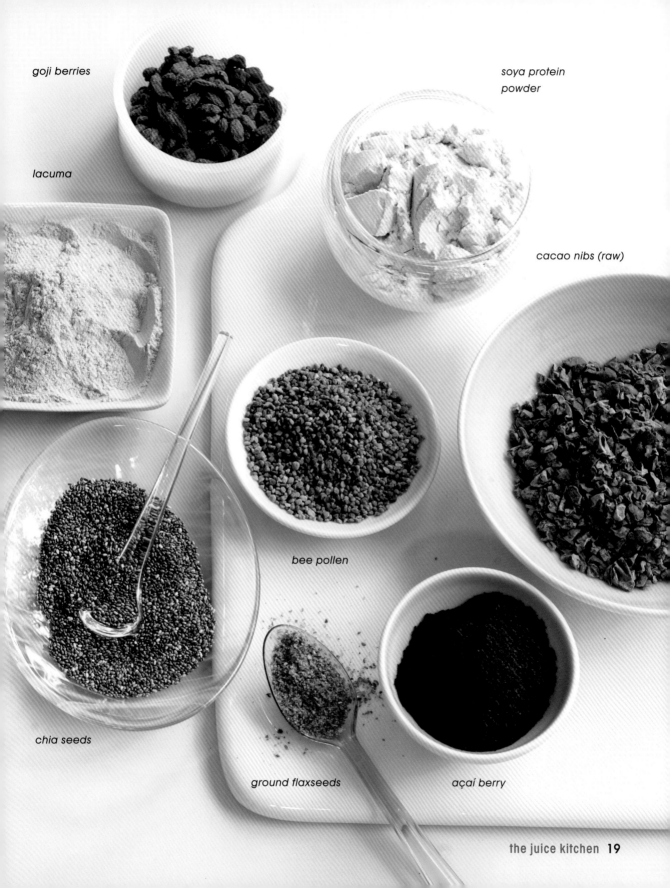

goji berries

soya protein powder

lacuma

cacao nibs (raw)

bee pollen

chia seeds

ground flaxseeds

açaí berry

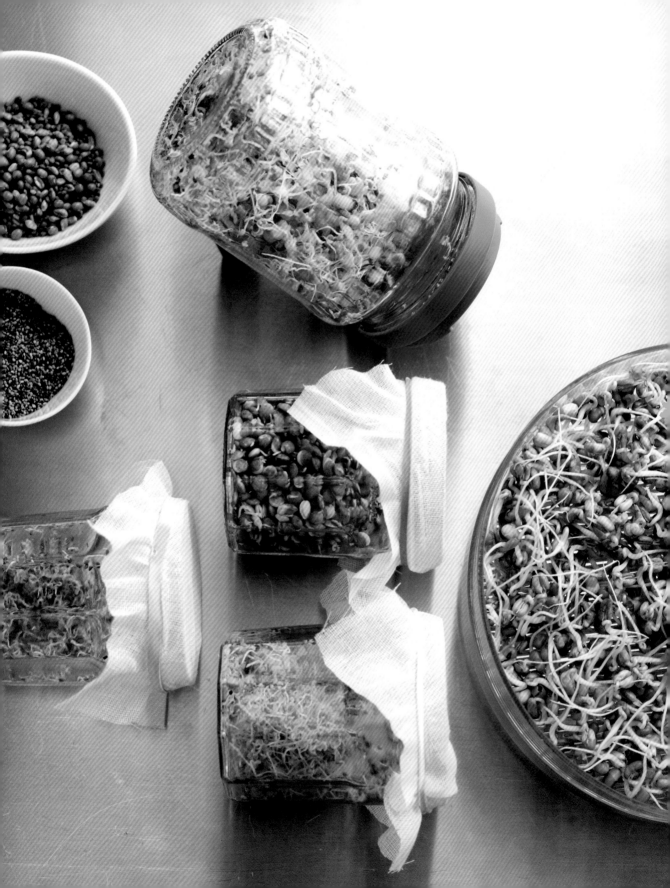

Sprout-your-own seeds

Seeds, beans and grains can all be sprouted and are easy to grow at home without any specialist equipment.

Fresh sprouted seeds, beans and grains are super healthy as their nutritional value jumps dramatically when germinated. In their sprouted form they provide around 30 per cent more B vitamins and 60 per cent more vitamin C than in the dormant seed, pulse or grain. They are also rich in protein, vitamins A, D, E and K as well as the minerals iron, zinc, calcium, magnesium, selenium and potassium. In Chinese medicine they are highly valued for their ability to cleanse and rejuvenate the body.

The choice of seeds to buy for sprouting is incredible, from the ubiquitous alfalfa, which is probably the easiest to grow, to vegetable seeds such as the potent, cancer-preventing broccoli and radish. There are herb seeds including chives and parsley, grain seeds such as buckwheat, which is good for the digestion and circulation, and rejuvenating flaxseeds, renowned for their high omega-3 fatty acid content and cholesterol-lowering properties. Look, too, for seed mixes, which have often been carefully blended to suit particular health requirements, such as a detox blend, fitness blend or good health blend.

The choice of protein and mineral-rich beans and pulses for sprouting is equally diverse, including the ever-popular mung beansprout, a mainstay in Asian cooking; the wispy, white sprouts of the aduki bean; peppery and slightly spicy lentil sprouts and the nutty, substantial chickpea sprout.

Seed, bean and grain sprouts are living foods and are most nutritionally potent when eaten raw (or very lightly cooked), meaning they are perfect in smoothies and blends. They can be juiced, though admittedly they don't provide much in the way of liquid and you will probably need to help them through the juicer by interspersing them with juicier fruit or vegetables. If your appliance is able to juice wheatgrass, then it will no doubt be able to deal with sprouts.

A jam jar, a piece of muslin/cheesecloth and an elastic band are all you need to get sprouting but regular, keen sprouters or those who like to sprout different types of seeds at a time may like to invest in specialist kit. When I say specialist, a sprouter unit is pretty basic and reasonably priced, made up of stacking (and draining) trays. The trays allow ventilation, which help prevent mould growth.

How to sprout seeds

1 *To sprout seeds in a jar, rinse around 3 tablespoons of seeds thoroughly in water, then place in a bowl. Pour over lukewarm water until well covered, put a plate on top and leave to stand overnight.*

2 *The next day, drain the seeds, rinse and drain again, then tip them into a large, clean jar. Cover with a double piece of muslin/cloth, held in place with an elastic band. Put the jar on its side in a warm place away from direct sunlight.*

3 *Rinse the seeds 2–4 times a day, draining thoroughly each time to prevent them turning mouldy; you don't want them to be completely dry. The seed pack will advise on rinsing and sprouting times, but seeds usually take around 3–10 days, depending on the variety. After 2 days, you can move the jars into direct sunlight to encourage the chlorophyll and increase the sprouts' magnesium and fibre content.*

4 *When about 2.5–5 cm/1–2 inches in length, tip the sprouts out of the jar and discard any that haven't sprouted, transfer them to a lidded container and store in the fridge for up to 3 days.*

Make-your-own nut milks

Homemade nut milks are easy to make. Almond and cashew nut milks are both favourites, or you could try hazelnut, pistachio, peanut, walnut, Brazil or macadamia. Sunflower or pumpkin seed milk is also an option, as is oat milk.

Simply soak the nuts in pure or filtered water overnight at room temperature then drain, rinse and blend with fresh pure or filtered water. The resulting milky liquid then needs to be strained through a nut bag or piece of muslin. Don't waste the nut meal left in the nut bag or muslin/cloth as it can be used in smoothies or to make granola, muesli or cookies, or even dehydrated into flour. Some say the initial soaking of the nuts isn't strictly necessary as they can be blended straightaway in water but it produces a creamier end result. Also, since some nuts contain enzyme inhibitors, which make it difficult for the body to absorb their nutrients, it makes sense to soak them.

This recipe uses three times the quantity of pure or filtered water to nuts for an everyday but still rich milk, but you can reduce the quantity of water to make a thicker milk or even a cream substitute. You can sweeten the milk with honey, dates, agave or maple syrup, but it is just as good unadulterated. A sprinkling of ground cinnamon or nutmeg and a splash of vanilla extract make delicious additions, too.

If you regularly make nut milks it may be worth a small investment in a nut milk bag, which makes straining and draining the nuts from the milk that much easier; and you can also use it for sprouting seeds.

How to make almond milk

150 g/1 cup shelled almonds
750 ml/3 cups pure or filtered water,
 plus extra for soaking

1 *Put the almonds in a large bowl and cover with about 2.5 cm/1 inch pure or filtered water. Cover with a plate and leave to stand overnight. The next day, drain the almonds and rinse them under cold running water.*

2 *Put the soaked almonds in a blender with the 750 ml/3 cups pure or filtered water and blend on a high speed for about 2 minutes, or until the nuts are broken down into a fine meal and the water is creamy white.*

3 *Strain the almonds through a nut milk bag or a muslin-lined/cheesecloth-lined sieve, reserving the strained milky liquid in a bowl. Gather up the sides of the bag or the muslin/cloth in the sieve and squeeze to extract as much liquid as possible into the bowl containing the milky liquid. Pour the milk into a lidded container or bottle and store in the fridge up to 3 days. The nut meal left in the bag or muslin/cloth can be used as instructed on the left.*

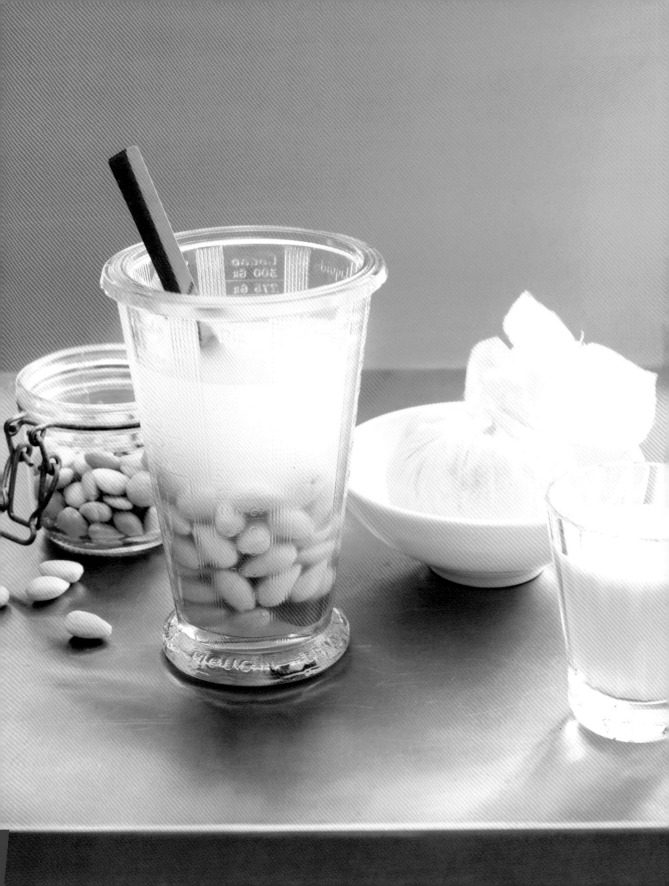

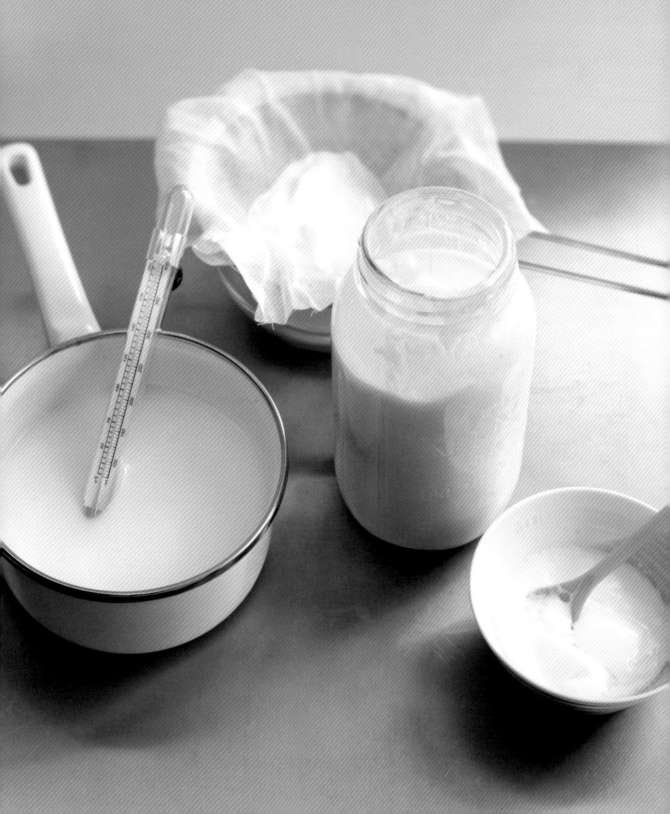

Make-your-own yogurt

Yogurt is immensely rewarding to make and once you've made your first batch of yogurt, you can reserve a portion of it to use as a starter for the next; just make sure you use live yogurt for your starter and it's very fresh.

'Live' on the label signifies a yogurt that has been fermented with a starter culture bacteria, such as *lactobacillus acidophilus*. The beneficial bacteria in live or bio yogurt helps to restore the internal flora of the gut by encouraging 'friendly' bacteria, aiding digestion and gastrointestinal problems and suppressing the effects of 'bad' bacteria. Yogurt is also a good source of calcium and B vitamins.

A special yogurt maker isn't necessary here, but you will need a kitchen thermometer and a mason or screw-top jar. It's also important to be scrupulous about hygiene, so make sure your equipment is sterilized before you start.

Depending on what time of year you make yogurt, you will need to consider how to keep it warm while it cultures. In hot, sunny weather, wrap the jar in layers of towels and a black plastic bag and this should be sufficient to keep the contents warm, while in the colder winter months a thermos flask, warm airing cupboard or an oven heated to 100°F/38°C are possible alternatives.

How to make live yogurt

This recipe makes about 1 litre/1 quart of fresh-tasting, light yogurt, which is perfect in smoothies and lassies, but you could use a whole milk yogurt for a creamier, richer end result. Instead of cow's milk, sheep's or goats' milk are both options.

1 litre/4 cups organic semi-skimmed/low-fat milk
3 tablespoons organic plain live yogurt

1 *Pour the milk into a large, heavy-based saucepan and bring slowly to boiling point over a medium-low heat, stirring occasionally to prevent the milk burning on the bottom of the pan; it should read 185°F/85°C on a kitchen thermometer. Once the milk has reached this heat, keep it there for about 10 minutes, stirring occasionally. You may need to turn the heat down to low during this time.*

2 *Turn the heat off, remove any skin that has formed on the surface of the milk and leave the mixture to cool to 110°F/43°C, uncovered and stirring occasionally. This usually takes around 40–45 minutes.*

3 *Spoon the live yogurt into a 1-litre mason or screw-top jar/a 4-cup sterilizing canning jar and pour in a quarter of the warm milk. Stir well until combined, then add the remaining milk and stir again. Fasten the lid and wrap the jar in clingfilm/plastic wrap, towels and then a black plastic bag to keep the warmth in.*

4 *Leave the jar a warm place, ideally around 100°F/38°C, for 8 hours or overnight until set. Alternatively, transfer the milk mixture to a warmed Thermos flask and leave for 8 hours or overnight until set. When ready, stir well and chill in the fridge until ready to eat; it will thicken up a bit more as it cools. If you want a Greek-style yogurt, line a sieve with a double layer of muslin/cheesecloth and strain the yogurt over a bowl in the fridge for about 1 hour until it is thick and creamy; the whey in the bowl can be used in smoothies and blends. Store the yogurt in the fridge for up to 1 week.*

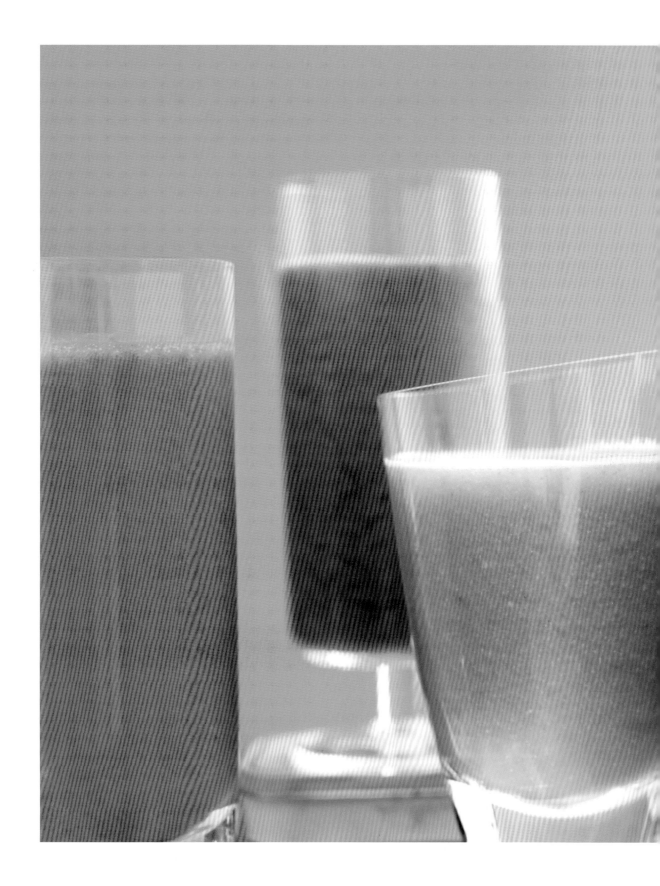

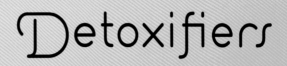

Detoxifiers

Virgin apple mojito

I love the hit from the lime juice and fresh mint in this vibrantly green, zingy juice. This makes a refreshing, cooling drink served on ice or you could top it up with chilled carbonated mineral water. If serving this to non-vegetable lovers, you'd never know the kale was there!

4 medium green apples, quartered,
   cored and cut into wedges
2 large handfuls of curly kale
1 handful of fresh mint
juice of ½–1 lime
1–2 teaspoons barleygrass powder (*see page 14*)
crushed ice, to serve

SERVES 2

Juice the apples, kale and three-quarters of the mint – add a splash of the lime juice if the juicer struggles with the kale. Stir the lime juice and barleygrass into the juice and serve on crushed ice. Chop the reserved mint leaves and sprinkle over the top.

Super detox

Lemon not only adds a real lift to the flavour of this cleansing juice but it also stops it oxidising, helping to retain its colour and nutrients. Wheatgrass, barleygrass or spirulina can all be used instead of the chlorella.

2 pears, quartered and cored
1 celery stick
1 handful of spinach
2 large handfuls of curly kale
½ large cucumber, quartered lengthways
juice of 1 lemon
1–2 teaspoons chlorella powder (*see page 15*)

SERVES 2

Juice the pears, celery, spinach, kale and cucumber. Stir in the lemon juice and chlorella until combined.

> **kale** is one of the healthiest vegetables around and has been shown to actively help the body's detoxification system. Like its fellow cruciferous vegetables, including cabbage and broccoli, it is recommended that you eat kale 2–3 times a week for optimum anti-inflammatory, antioxidant and anti-cancer benefits. It also is a good source of vitamins A, C, K and B6.

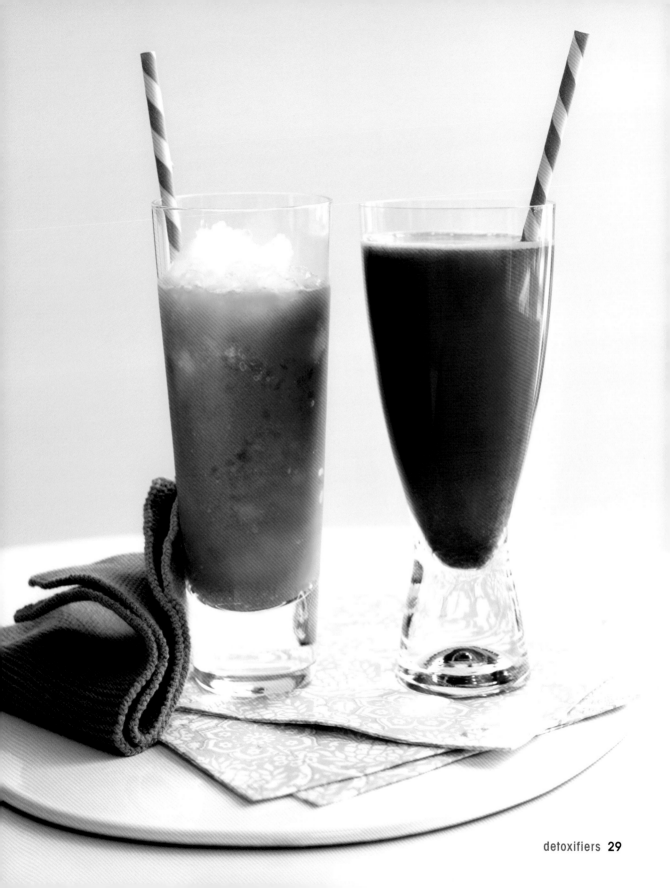

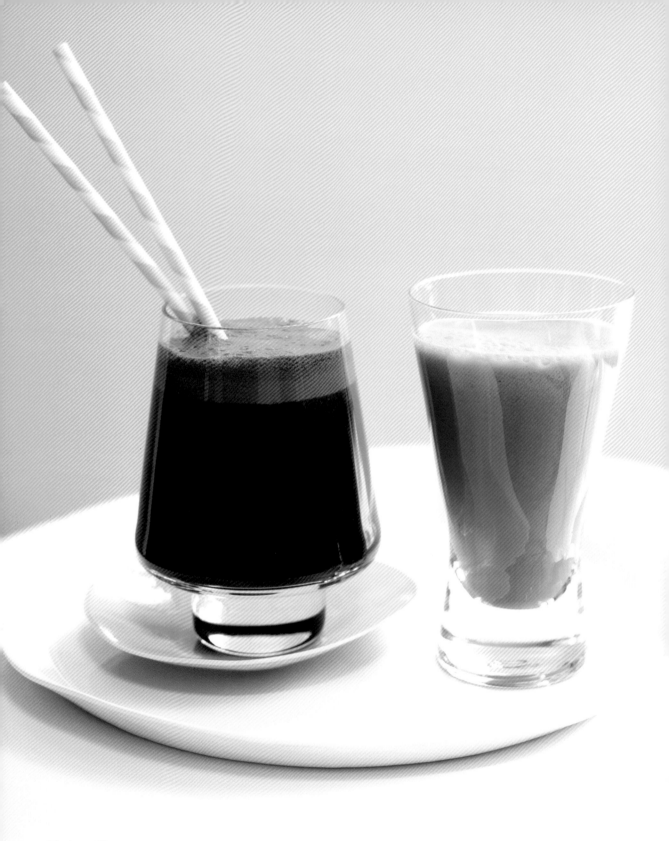

Deep purple

The beetroot/beets and red cabbage give a pleasant earthiness to this juice, which is lifted by the sweetness of the grapes. It has an amazing colour, too! Check the daily dosage on your bottle of milk thistle extract as the recommended amount can vary depending on the brand.

2 carrots, peeled and halved lengthways

2 raw beetroot/beets, quartered

2 handfuls of sliced red cabbage

5 radishes, halved

3 large handfuls of seedless black grapes

2 teaspoons spirulina powder (*see page 18*)

6–12 drops milk thistle extract (*see page 18*)
  (check the recommended dosage on the bottle)

SERVES 2

Juice the carrots, beetroot/beets, red cabbage, radishes and grapes then stir in the spirulina and milk thistle.

Apple zinger

Simplicity in a glass – fresh root ginger gives a real zing to this juice and is just the thing to revive you after long night! Apple lends a touch of sweetness and helps to balance out the earthiness of the spinach.

4 apples, quartered, cored and cut into wedges

2.5-cm/1-inch piece fresh root ginger, unpeeled

2 large handfuls of spinach

1 teaspoon lemon juice

1 teaspoon powdered greens mix (*see page 17*)

1 teaspoon wheatgrass powder (*see page 18*)

SERVES 2

Juice the apples, ginger and spinach then stir in the lemon juice, greens and wheatgrass.

ginger has a settling affect on the stomach and can reduce nausea. It also has painkilling, antibacterial and anti-inflammatory benefits, while spinach is packed with nutrients such as vitamins A, B, C, E and K as well as iron, magnesium and calcium. Iron is more readily absorbed when eaten in conjunction with vitamin C-rich foods such as the apples used here.

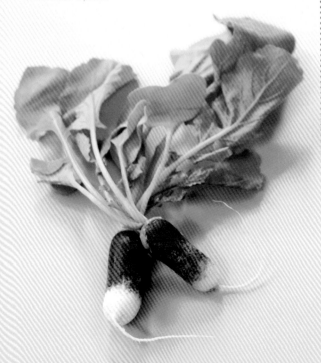

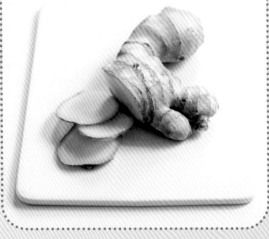

Minty fresh

Fresh juices are easy to digest, helping to flush out the digestive system and encourage the elimination of toxins. Carrot, pear, grape, lemon and mint are a great combination and all are said to be effective detoxifiers.

6 medium carrots,
   peeled and halved lengthways
4 just-ripe pears,
   quartered and cored lengthways
2 good handfuls of white seedless grapes
juice of 1 small lemon
1 teaspoon chopped mint leaves
chia seeds, for sprinkling (*see page 15*)

SERVES 2

Juice the carrots, pears and grapes and stir in the lemon juice and mint. Sprinkle with chia seeds before serving.

Green giant

Not for the faint-hearted – you just know that this intensely green juice is doing you good! Choose watercress sold loose in bundles for the best flavour and nutrient value.

1 chilled cucumber, quartered lengthways

3 handfuls of watercress

1 head of broccoli, both florets and stalks, chopped

juice of ½ lemon

½ teaspoon extra virgin olive oil

1–2 teaspoons wheatgrass powder (*see page 18*)

SERVES 2–3

Juice the cucumber, watercress (if your machine struggles with the watercress, add a splash of water or some of the lemon juice), broccoli florets and stalks. Stir in the lemon juice, olive oil and wheatgrass.

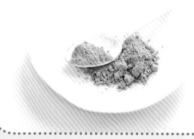

wheatgrass is a powerful detoxifier, blood-purifier and cleanser. Partnered with watercress and broccoli, this juice provides an impressive catalogue of nutrients, antioxidants and phytonutrients.

An apple a day...

Apples are a common feature in many detox diets and for good reason. They are particularly effective in removing impurities from the liver and, like carrots, are a good source of the antioxidant, beta-carotene.

2 medium apples, quartered, cored and cut into wedges
5 medium carrots, peeled and halved lengthways
2 large uncooked beetroot/beets, peeled and cut into wedges
juice of 1 small lemon
1–2 teaspoons wheatgrass powder *(see page 18)*

SERVES 2

Juice the apples, carrots and beetroot/beets then stir in the lemon juice and wheatgrass powder.

Big purple cleanse

A great liver cleanser, this juice also tastes good with the spicy tang of the red cabbage and earthiness of the beetroot/beet balanced out by the sweetness of the grapes.

6 handfuls of sliced red cabbage
3 medium uncooked beetroot/beets
6 handfuls of black seedless grapes
½–1 teaspoon chlorella powder *(see page 15)*

SERVES 2

Juice the red cabbage, beetroot/beets and grapes then stir in the chlorella.

black grapes Effective as part of a detox diet, grapes also help to treat skin conditions, gout and liver and kidney disorders. What's more, studies show that grape juice from black grapes is said to be as effective as aspirin in reducing the risk of heart attacks.

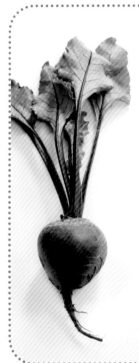

beetroot/beet
A juice to drink on a regular basis, beetroot/beet is recommended as a daily tonic. Beetroot/beets contain calcium, iron, beta-carotene and vitamin C and is an effective detoxifier and laxative. It's also good for treating and preventing anaemia, so this is a great juice for women.

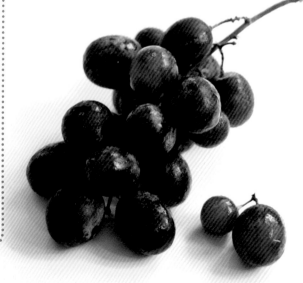

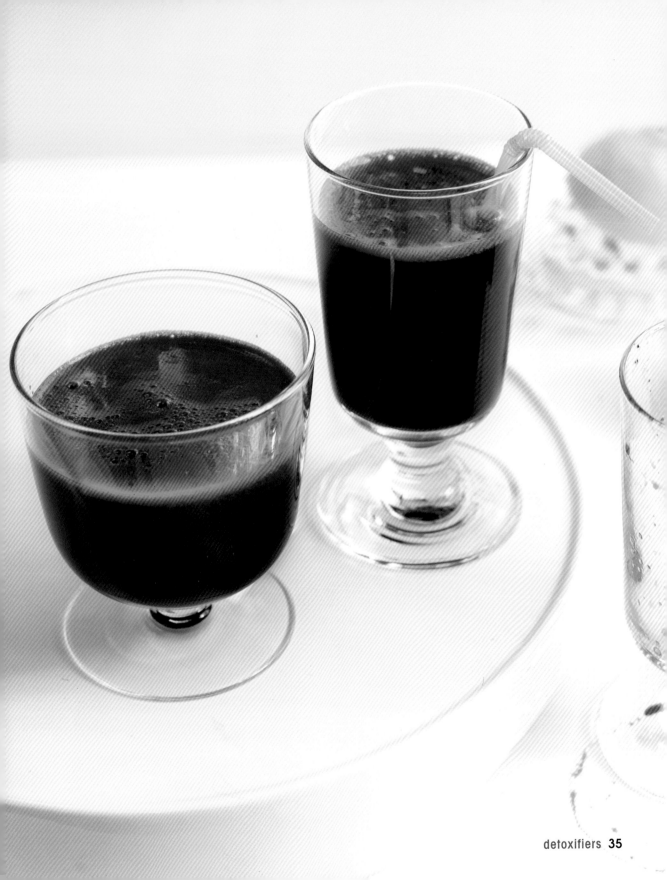

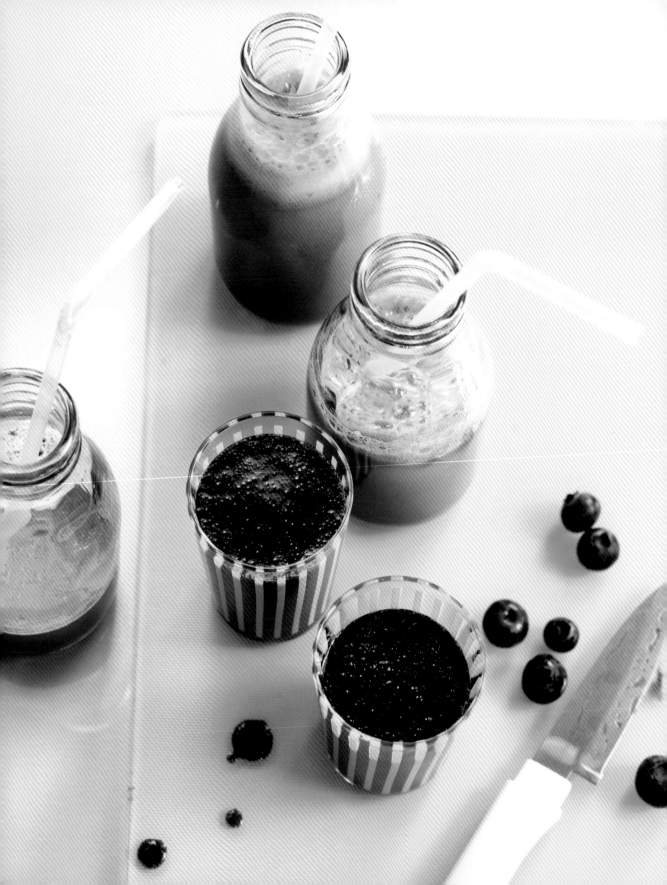

Deep cleanser

Strawberries make a surprisingly rich and creamy juice and, thanks to the presence of the powerful antioxidant ellagic acid, encourage liver-cleansing enzymes to escort toxins out of the body, particularly those linked with causing cancer.

4 handfuls of strawberries, hulled

3 handfuls of spinach leaves

2 handfuls of blueberries

1 large uncooked beetroot/beet, peeled and cut into wedges

2.5-cm/1-inch piece fresh root ginger, peeled and halved

juice of 1 lemon

1 teaspoon açaí berry powder *(see page 14)*

1–2 teaspoons detox greens powder *(see page 16)*

SERVES 2

Juice the strawberries, spinach, blueberries, beetroot and ginger then stir in the lemon juice, açaí berry powder and detox greens mixture.

> **strawberries** Alongside their liver-cleansing capabilities, strawberries are rich in B vitamins and vitamin C as well as the mineral potassium, which helps to maintain normal blood pressure and supports the kidneys.

Green shot

The vitamin C in the lemon helps the absorption of the iron provided by the spinach and parsley. Iron is an important mineral and aids detoxification that takes place in the liver.

4 handfuls of spinach

2 handfuls of parsley

4 handfuls of watercress

3 medium apples, quartered, cored and cut into wedges

2.5-cm/1-inch piece fresh root ginger, peeled and halved

juice of 1 lemon

1–2 teaspoons wheatgrass powder *(see page 18)*

SERVES 2

Juice the spinach, parsley and watercress, interspersing them with wedges of apple to help them through the juicer, then juice the ginger and stir in the lemon juice and wheatgrass.

> **watercress** The super-nutrient PEITC found naturally in watercress and also in broccoli, cauliflower and cabbage has been found to cleanse and protect the lungs from pollution and cigarette smoke as well as reduce the risk of certain forms of cancer, including ovarian.

Eye eye

Carrots aren't just great for vision, they also help to cleanse, nourish and stimulate the whole body. As well as being nutritionally generous, they also provide a lot of liquid when juiced as well as a slight sweetness.

6 medium carrots, peeled and halved lengthways
4 handfuls of shredded white cabbage
2 medium pears, quartered and cored
2.5-cm/1-inch piece fresh root ginger, peeled and halved
1–2 teaspoons detox mix (see page 16)
chia seeds, for sprinkling

SERVES 2

Juice the carrots, white cabbage, pears and ginger then stir in the detox mix and sprinkle with chia seeds before serving.

Spring clean

Don't waste the stalks from the broccoli as they are just as good juiced as the florets. Providing a potent combination of super-nutrients, this fruit and vegetable juice is further enhanced by the green algae, chlorella.

3 good handfuls of broccoli, including stalks
4 medium apples, quartered, cored and cut into wedges
4 handfuls of spinach
1 celery stick
4 handfuls of shredded spring greens
juice of 1 lime
1–2 teaspoons chlorella powder (see page 15)

SERVES 2

Juice the broccoli, apples, spinach, celery and spring greens then stir in the lime juice and chlorella.

broccoli Along with other brassicas, broccoli contains the super antioxidant glutathione, which cleanses and protects the liver from damage as it processes pollutants and toxins.

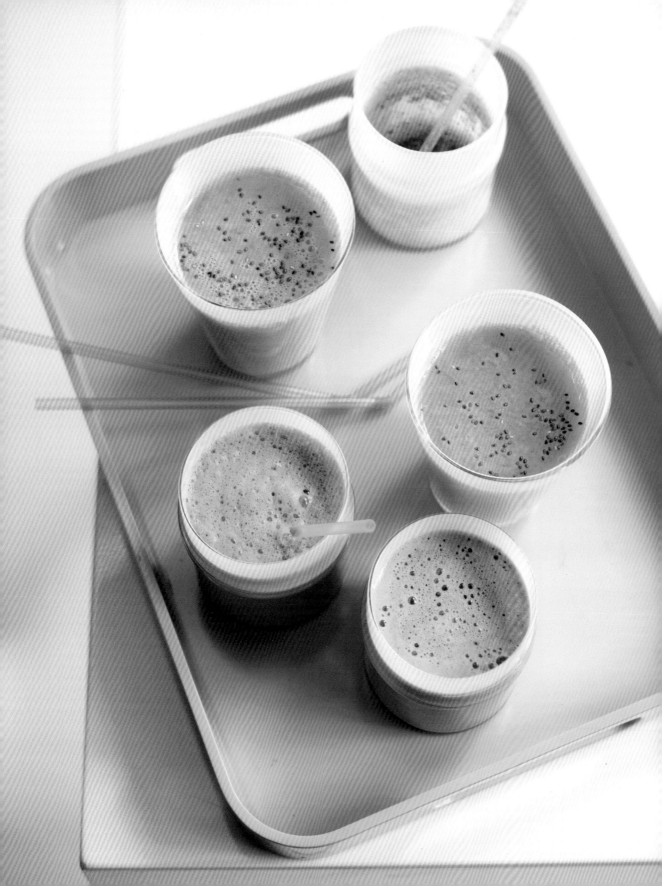

Carrot and garlic smoopie

A cross between a soup and a smoothie, this is a perfect meal substitute if following a detox plan. The sulphur compounds in garlic help to get rid of unwanted toxins as well as bacteria and parasites from the colon.

Put the carrots, red pepper, tomatoes, parsley, garlic, radish sprouts, flaxseeds, turmeric and lemon juice in a blender. Add 250 ml/1 cup pure or filtered water and the barleygrass powder and blend until smooth. Add a splash more water if too thick.

2 carrots, peeled and chopped

1 large red (bell) pepper, deseeded and chopped

2 good-size vine-ripened tomatoes, chopped

1 handful of flat-leaf parsley

2 small garlic cloves, peeled

1 handful of radish sprouts (see page 21)

2 teaspoons ground flaxseeds (see page 16)

¼ teaspoon ground turmeric

juice of 1 lemon

1–2 teaspoons barleygrass powder (see page 14)

SERVES 2

Green day

Brassicas such as broccoli, cabbage and kale contain nutrients that boost the liver enzyme called glutathione, which helps to cleanse the liver of heavy metals.

1 green apple, cut into wedges and cored
4 broccoli florets
1 handful of rocket/arugula leaves
½ cucumber, peeled, deseeded and cut into pieces
juice of ½ lemon
250 ml/1 cup coconut water
1–2 teaspoons wheatgrass powder (*see page 18*)

SERVES 2

Put the apple, broccoli, rocket/arugula, cucumber, lemon juice, coconut water and wheatgrass powder in a blender and blend until smooth. Add a splash of pure or filtered water if too thick.

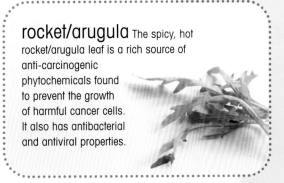

rocket/arugula The spicy, hot rocket/arugula leaf is a rich source of anti-carcinogenic phytochemicals found to prevent the growth of harmful cancer cells. It also has antibacterial and antiviral properties.

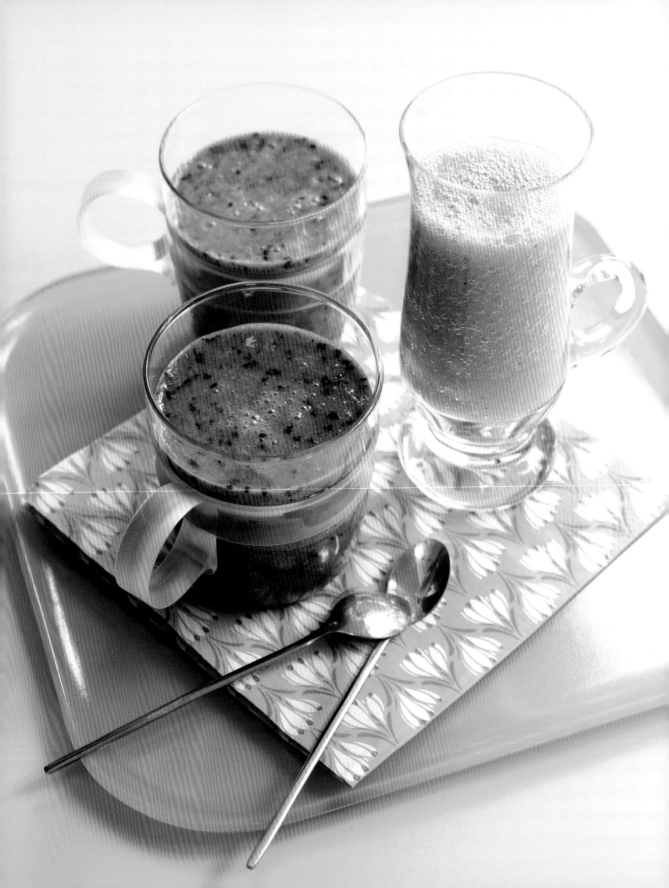

Clear mind

Blueberries are not only delicious juiced, they have also been shown to increase blood flow to the brain, clearing the mind and boosting memory and concentration.

2 handfuls of chopped, peeled sweet potato
2 handfuls of blueberries
400 ml/1⅔ cups freshly squeezed orange juice
juice of ½ lemon
2 teaspoons açaí berry powder *(see page 14)*
1–2 teaspoons chlorella powder *(see page 15)*

SERVES 2

Put the sweet potato, blueberries, orange and lemon juices, açaí berry and chlorella powders in a blender and blend until smooth. Add more orange juice if needed.

blueberries One of the few fruits to give us both vitamin C and E, this combo is great for detoxing the skin and helping to protect it against sun damage.

Pear chai

Spices not only enhance flavour, they are great for the digestive system. Cinnamon is an effective detoxifier and cleanser and, like many spices, has antibacterial properties.

4 ripe pears, peeled, cored and chopped
300 ml/1¼ cups white tea, cooled
1 tablespoon lemon juice
seeds from 2–3 cardamom pods, ground
½ teaspoon ground cinnamon
4-cm/1½-inch piece fresh root ginger,
   peeled and finely grated
few drops milk thistle *(see page 18)*
   (check the recommended dosage on the bottle)

SERVES 2

Put the pears, white tea, lemon juice, ground cardamom and cinnamon in a blender. Squeeze the juice from the grated ginger through your fingers and add to the blender, then blend until smooth. Stir in the milk thistle drops.

white tea Research shows that white tea is even better for us than green with a higher proportion of the antioxidant polyphenols that destroy cancer-causing cells. The young tea leaves also have antibacterial properties, helping to boost the immune system.

Sleep easy

You may be asleep but your body is busy repairing and maintaining itself, so help it on its way with this calming drink. Camomile and lettuce are recognised for their soporific qualities, helping you to sleep well and in turn enhance the detoxing process.

2 camomile tea bags

4 handfuls of white, seedless grapes

2 handfuls of soft leaf lettuce

juice of 1 large lemon

4-cm/½-inch piece fresh root ginger, peeled and
   finely grated

few drops milk thistle (*see page 18*)
   (*check the recommended dosage on the bottle*)

SERVES 2

Make the camomile tea with 500 ml/2 cups boiled water and allow to steep for 5 minutes. Remove the tea bags and allow to cool. Pour the cooled camomile tea into a blender and add the grapes, lettuce and lemon juice. Squeeze the juice from the grated ginger through your fingers and add to the blender, then blend until smooth. Stir in the milk thistle and drink before bedtime for a restful night's sleep.

In the red

The popular South African tea, rooibos (red bush), makes a great fruity base for this blended juice and is also good for you, being rich in antioxidants, caffeine-free and low in tannins, which inhibit the absorption of valuable minerals such as iron.

300 ml/1¼ cups rooibos tea, cooled

2 medium apples, peeled, cored and chopped

1 medium beetroot/beet, peeled and chopped

1.5-cm/⅝-inch piece fresh root ginger, peeled and
   finely grated

1–2 teaspoons wheatgrass powder (*see page 18*)

SERVES 2

Put the cooled rooibos tea, apples and beetroot/beet in a blender. Squeeze the juice from the grated ginger through your fingers and add to the blender with the wheatgrass, then blend until smooth.

lettuce Although 95 per cent water, lettuce is surprisingly nutritious as well as cleansing. A mild diuretic, lettuce contains significant amounts of folic acid, vitamin C and potassium and is also a general tonic for the digestive system and skin.

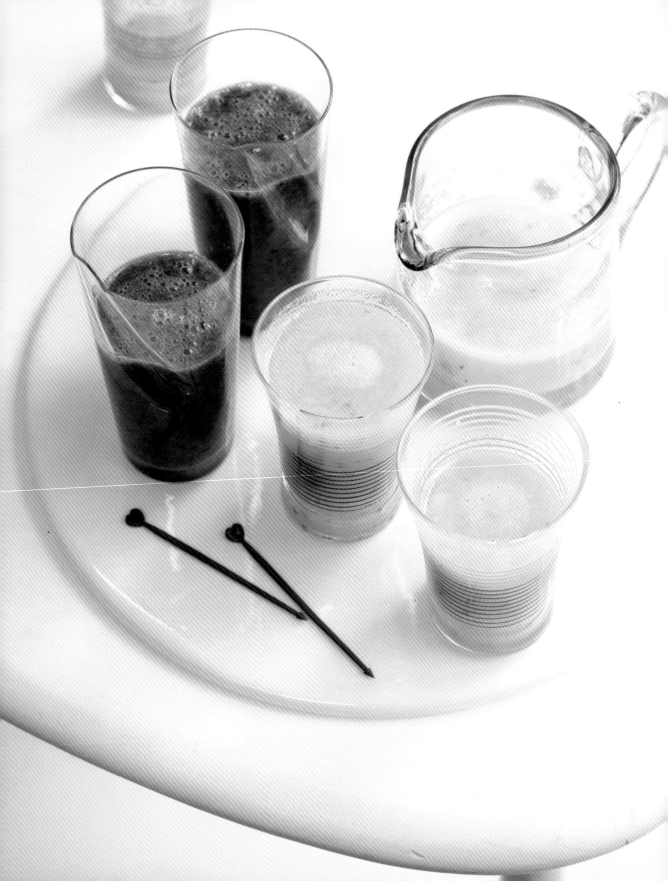

Feeling flush

Prunes lend a rich, sweetness to this drink, but their real claim to fame is their ability to prevent constipation and improve the intestinal flora of the digestive system. The cleansing prunes are further boosted by the kale, orange juice and spirulina.

10 ready-to-eat dried pitted prunes, halved
2 handfuls kale, tough stalks discarded,
   leaves shredded
1 small handful of alfalfa sprouts (*see page 21*)
300 ml/1¼ cups freshly squeezed orange juice
juice of ½ lemon
1–2 teaspoons spirulina (*see page 18*)

SERVES 2

Put the prunes, kale, alfalfa, orange juice, lemon juice and spirulina in a blender with 100 ml/ ⅓ cup pure or filtered water, then blend until smooth. Add a splash more water if it is too thick.

Lemon detox

Knock this back first thing to give your body a kick start and help an overworked liver. You could add super-hydrating coconut water instead of pure or filtered water.

1 apple, cored and chopped
juice of 1 large lemon
¼ teaspoon cayenne pepper
1–2 teaspoons detox greens powder (*see page 16*)
few drops milk thistle (*see page 18*)
   (*check the recommended dosage on the bottle*)

SERVES 2

Put the apple, lemon juice, cayenne pepper, detox greens and milk thistle in a blender with 300 ml/ 1¼ cups pure or filtered water. Blend until smooth.

cayenne pepper
This fiery red powder has effective antiseptic and digestive qualities. It is a powerful stimulant, helping to improve and boost blood circulation.

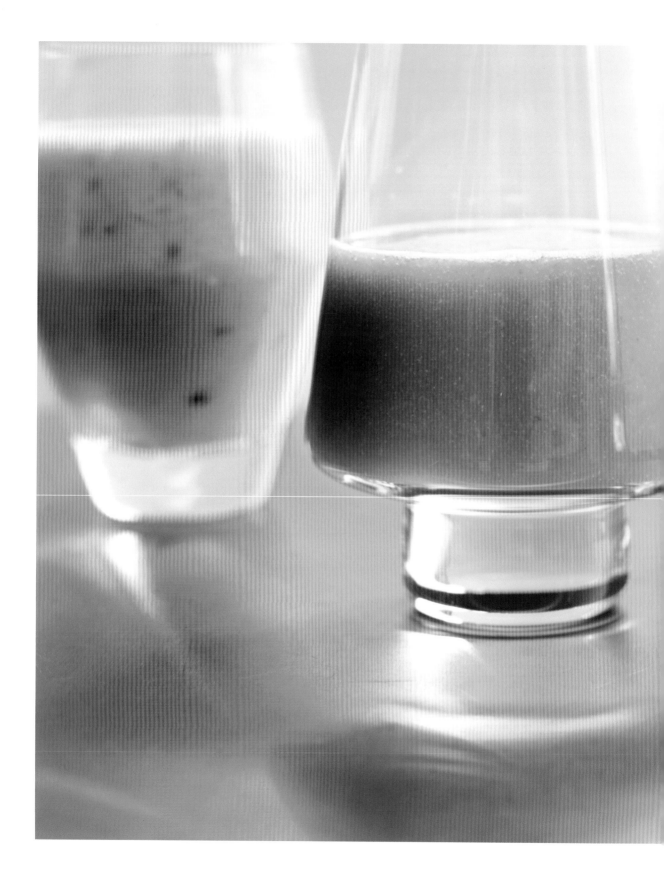

Energy-enhancers

Good morning

When you know your iron levels are lacking and you're feeling below par, then start the day with this iron-rich, reviving juice for a week or two.

2 large oranges, peeled and quartered
2 medium uncooked beetroot/beets, peeled and quartered
2 medium carrots, peeled and halved lengthways
1 good handful of seedless black grapes
1 teaspoon lemon juice
2 teaspoons açaí berry powder (*see page 14*)
¼ teaspoon chia seeds (*see page 15*)

SERVES 2

chia seeds despite their diminutive size pack a powerful nutritional punch. Classified as a complete protein, they contain all the essential amino acids and are also a rich plant source of omega-3 fatty acids.

Juice the oranges, beetroot/beets, carrots and grapes then stir in the lemon juice and açaí powder. Sprinkle with the chia seeds.

Popeye special

Spinach contains decent amounts of iron but it's essential to eat a food rich in vitamin C at the same time to help the body absorb the mineral. Thankfully, fresh orange provides heaps of vitamin C as well as a refreshing zesty tang to this juice.

6 medium oranges, peeled and quartered
4 handfuls of spinach
4 handfuls of chopped pointed cabbage
150 ml/²⁄₃ cup green tea, cooled
6 basil leaves, chopped
1 teaspoon finely grated orange zest

SERVES 2

Juice the oranges, spinach and cabbage and stir in the cooled green tea and basil leaves. Serve sprinkled with orange zest.

Sunrise

Fresh mango and banana add a rich taste of the tropics to this energy-giving drink, while the star anise lends a delicious warmth and aroma. Bananas are a concentrated bundle of nutrients and their high starch content makes them a good source of sustained energy, but make sure you use them when ripe.

2 star anise
1 medium mango, peeled, pitted and chopped
juice of 1 large orange
1 medium carrot, peeled and coarsely grated
1 medium banana, peeled and chopped
2 teaspoons camu camu powder
   (see page 15)
ground nutmeg, for sprinkling
SERVES 2

Soak the star anise in 50 ml/3½ tablespoons just-boiled water overnight. Discard the star anise and put the mango and soaking water in a blender with the orange juice, carrot, banana and camu camu powder then blend until smooth. Add pure or filtered water if too thick and sprinkle with nutmeg just before serving.

Sweet friend

One of the richest plant sources of omega-3 fatty acids, flaxseed oil also increases the uptake of beta carotene from the sweet potatoes, (bell) pepper and beetroot/beets.

1 medium sweet potato, peeled and cut into long wedges

1 large red (bell) pepper, deseeded and cut into long wedges

1 medium uncooked beetroot/beet, peeled and cut into wedges

2 pears, cored and quartered

2.5-cm/1-inch piece fresh root ginger, peeled and halved

1 teaspoon flaxseed oil

1–2 teaspoons spirulina powder *(see page 18)*

SERVES 2

Juice the sweet potato, red (bell) pepper, beetroot/beet, pears and ginger and stir in the flaxseed oil and spirulina.

sweet potatoes

Look for orange-fleshed sweet potatoes, which have a higher nutritional content than the white-fleshed variety. A rich source of antioxidants, beta carotene and vitamin C, sweet potatoes also provide plentiful amounts of sustained energy and help to boost circulation.

Double coconut and blueberry boost

Described as the 'cure for all illnesses', fresh coconut has antibacterial, anti-parasitic and antifungal properties. It's also great for boosting energy levels so when combined with blueberries, apple and açaí berry powder this drink packs a powerful punch; drink for breakfast and you'll be ready to go!

coconut water from the inside of the coconut
2 small handfuls of freshly chopped coconut
2 handfuls of blueberries
2 apples, peeled, cored and chopped
juice of ½ lime
2 teaspoons açaí berry powder *(see page 14)*
SERVES 2

Prepare the fresh coconut by carefully banging a screwdriver into one of the 'eyes'. Pour the coconut water inside into a measuring jug/pitcher and top with pure or filtered water to make 300 ml/1¼ cups. Pour the coconut water into a blender. Using the back of a large blade, tap the circumference of the coconut to open it up. Scrape the fresh coconut out of the shell, the equivalent to 2 small handfuls, and add to the blender with the blueberries, apples, lime juice and açaí berry powder. Blend until almost smooth; there will be flecks of fresh coconut but if you want a smoother drink, blend again.

Melon reviver

Melon is easy to digest and so is good for providing an instant energy boost. Deliciously fruity, this vibrant juice is perfect for when you feel energy levels dropping mid afternoon.

1 cantaloupe melon, cut into thin wedges, skin and seeds removed
2 handfuls of strawberries, hulled
1 orange, peeled and quartered
2.5-cm/1-inch piece fresh root ginger, peeled and halved
1–2 teaspoons spirulina powder *(see page 18)*
bee pollen *(see page 15)*, for sprinkling
SERVES 2

Juice the melon, strawberries, orange and ginger and stir in the spirulina. Sprinkle with bee pollen before serving.

> **cantaloupe melon** is brimming with beta carotene and is a good source of vitamin C. It also contains the trace mineral silicon, which is crucial for maintaining healthy skin.

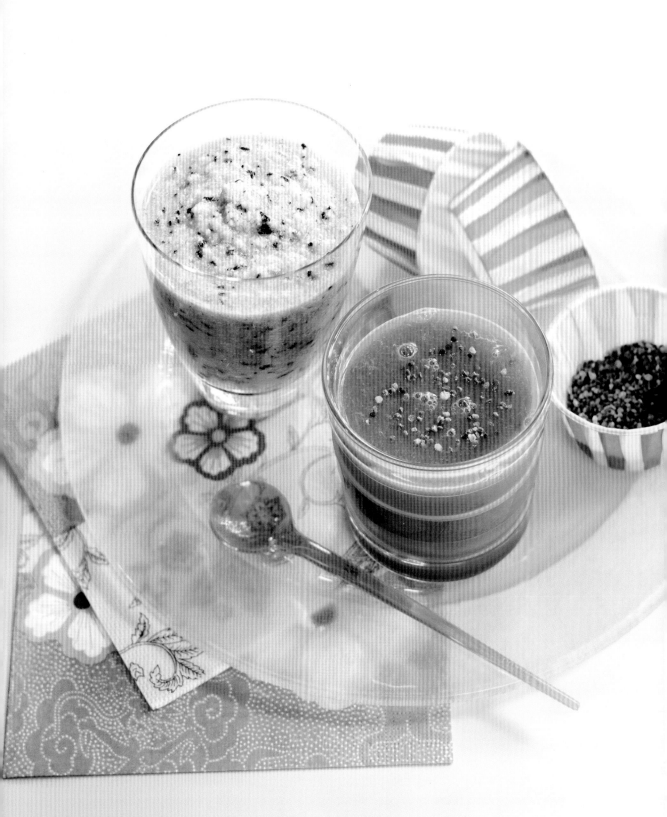

chillies/chiles are a powerful stimulant and expectorant and also have the reputation of being an aphrodisiac. Packed with vitamin C, they stimulate the release of endorphins, helping to lift mood and energy levels.

Rocket fuel

The chilli/chile certainly gives a kick to this nutrient-dense juice, which will liven you up for the day ahead. Remove the seeds from the chilli/chile if you prefer a tamer juice!

2 apples, quartered, cored and cut into wedges

2 large handfuls of curly kale

1 handful of broccoli, stalks and florets, chopped

2 medium carrots, peeled and halved lengthways

2 handfuls of alfalfa sprouts

1 medium red chilli/chile, quartered lengthways

2 teaspoons lemon juice

2 teaspoons powdered greens (*see page 17*)

1–2 teaspoons barleygrass (*see page 14*)

SERVES 2

Juice the apples, kale, broccoli, carrots, alfalfa sprouts and three-quarters of the chilli/chile. Stir in the lemon juice and powdered greens or barleygrass. Finely chop the reserved chilli/chile and sprinkle on top of each glass.

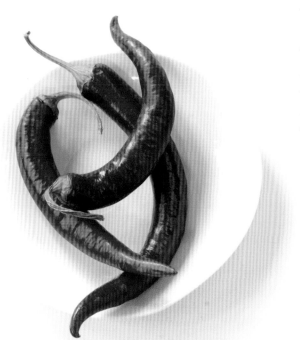

Super boost

Choose dark-coloured dried apricots if you can find them as they are not treated with the preservative sulphur, which has been linked to exacerbating the risk of an asthma attack in sufferers – they taste great too, adding an almost toffee-like quality to this immune-boosting juice.

5 unsulphured dried apricots

1 medium mango, peeled, pitted and sliced

2 large handfuls of strawberries

2 medium carrots, peeled and halved lengthways

1 tablespoon aloe vera juice (*see page 14*)

about 1 teaspoon probiotic powder (*see page 18*), (**check the recommended dosage on the bottle**)

SERVES 2

Soak the apricots in 100 ml/⅓ cup pure or filtered water for about 30 minutes (or overnight if making the juice the next morning) until softened. Juice the mango, strawberries, carrots, aloe vera and apricots, reserving the soaking water. Stir the probiotic powder into the soaking water, then add to the juice, stirring well until combined.

(You could blend this juice, but coarsely grate the carrots instead of cutting into slices. It will be slightly thicker in consistency so you may need to increase the quantity of water.)

Almond and date shake

Rich, creamy and sustaining, this is almost a meal in itself! Avocados are often misconstrued as being high in harmful fats and a food to avoid, but they are brimming with beneficial nutrients and the fat they contain is monounsaturated, which is believed to speed up the metabolic rate.

300 ml/1¼ cups almond milk *(see page 22)*,
   or milk of choice
3 handfuls of spinach, tough stalks discarded,
   shredded
1 small avocado, peeled, stoned and chopped
6 ready-to-eat dried dates, halved
2 teaspoons tahini paste
1–2 teaspoons barleygrass *(see page 14)*

SERVES 2

Put the almond milk, spinach, avocado, dates, tahini and barleygrass in a blender with 75 ml/scant ⅓ cup pure or filtered water and blend until smooth. Add more water if too thick.

Turbo tomato

Sun-dried tomatoes provide a concentrated unami, tomatoey flavour to this drink as well as a bundle of antioxidants, vitamins and minerals, especially B vitamins which are essential in converting food to energy.

4 sun-dried tomatoes (not in oil)
2 small handfuls of blanched almonds
2 tomatoes, chopped
2 medium carrots, peeled and coarsely grated
2 small handfuls of basil leaves, plus extra
   chopped for sprinkling
1 teaspoon ground flaxseeds *(see page 16)*
1–2 teaspoons açaí berry powder *(see page 14)*

SERVES 2

Soak the sun-dried tomatoes and almonds in 100 ml/⅓ cup just-boiled water for 1 hour, or overnight. Tip the sun-dried tomatoes, almonds and their soaking water into a blender and add the tomatoes, carrots, basil, ground flaxseeds and açaí berry powder. Pour in 225 ml/scant 1 cup pure or filtered water and blend until smooth. Serve sprinkled with extra basil.

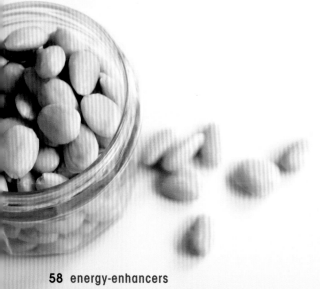

almonds In addition to B vitamins, vitamin E, calcium, magnesium and potassium, almonds are high in monounsaturated fats, the type that has been linked to a reduced risk of heart disease. B vitamins play an important role in energy production and may help prevent memory loss in later life.

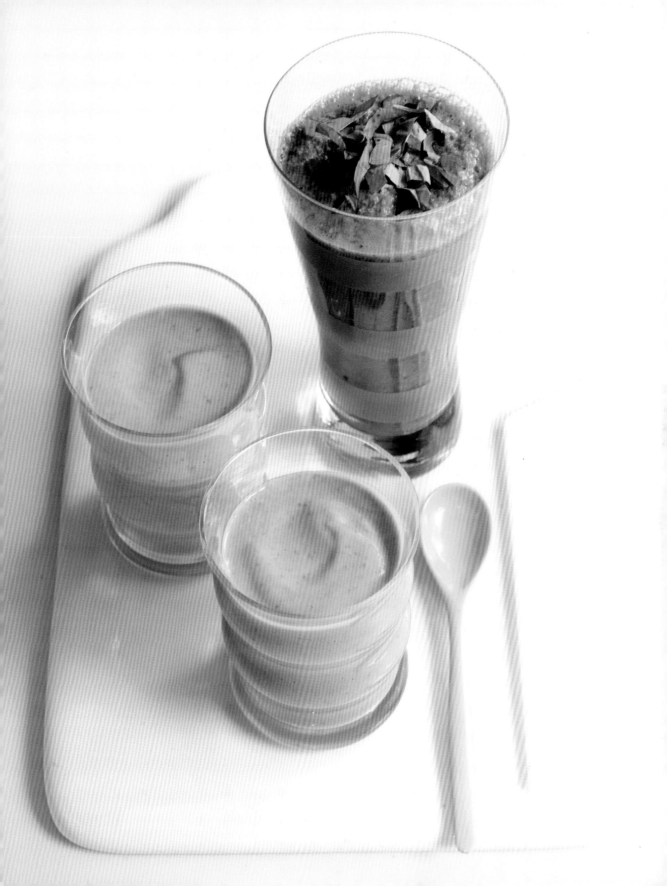

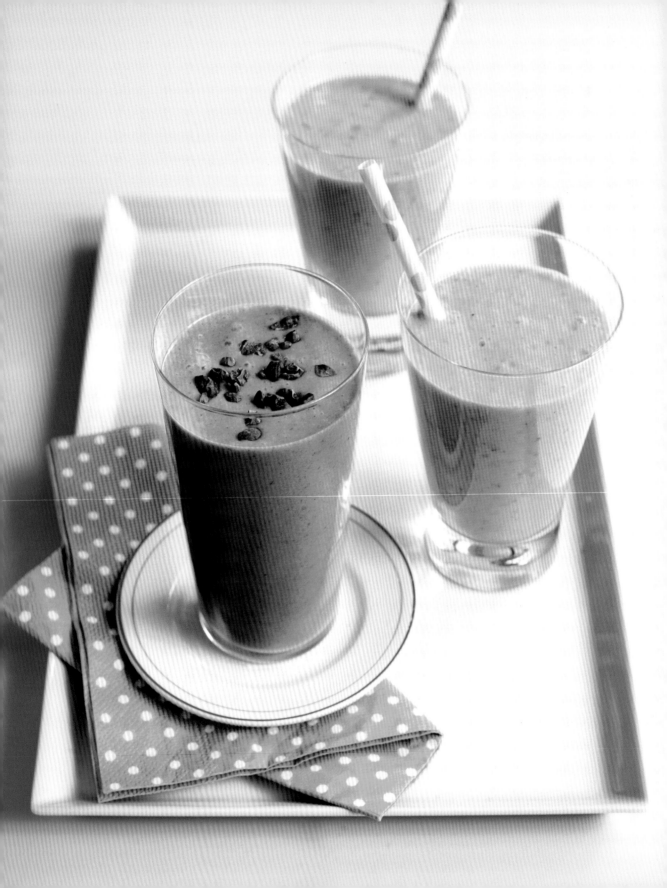

Choc-nut shake

The perfect sustaining breakfast in a glass for days when you don't have the stomach for something too substantial. Bananas provide an instant energy boost, while the malty-tasting maca is a potent combination of complex carbohydrates and protein. Try making your own almond milk, too.

250 ml/1 cup fresh almond milk (*see page 22*)
1 tablespoon smooth peanut butter
3 medium bananas, peeled and chopped
2 teaspoons maca powder (*see page 16*)
1 teaspoon raw cacao powder (*see page 15*)
½ teaspoon ground cinnamon
raw cacao nibs (*see page 15*), for sprinkling

SERVES 2

Put the almond milk, peanut butter, bananas, maca powder, raw cacao powder and cinnamon in a blender and blend until smooth. Serve sprinkled with the cacao nibs.

cinnamon is a wonderfully warming, nurturing spice with antioxidant and antimicrobial properties and is also said to help balance blood sugar levels. Maca, almonds and peanuts are a valuable source of brain-boosting, energy-giving protein.

bananas A concentrated bundle of energy, bananas are rich in potassium. This mineral aids the functioning of the body's cells, nerves and muscles as well as reducing high blood pressure and acting as an electrolyte.

Strawberries and cream

Strawberries and bananas are a classic smoothie combo, yet the old ones are the best! The addition of the superfood maca and ripe pear provide a nutritious twist.

200 ml/generous ¾ cup almond milk (*see page 22*), or milk of your choice
150 ml/⅔ cup plain bio yogurt
3 handfuls of strawberries, hulled
1 medium banana, peeled and chopped
1 medium pear, quartered, cored and chopped
½ teaspoon vanilla extract
½ teaspoon ground cinnamon, plus extra for sprinkling
2 teaspoons maca powder (*see page 16*)

SERVES 2

Put the almond milk, yogurt, strawberries, banana, pear, vanilla, cinnamon and maca in a blender and blend until smooth. Sprinkle with extra cinnamon, if desired.

Blackberry crumble

This reminds me of the traditional British crumble dessert, but served in a glass! Great for breakfast when time is against you and you're looking for nutritious sustenance for the day ahead, or why not serve it as a healthy dessert?

2 good handfuls of fresh or frozen blackberries
2 ripe pears, peeled, cored and roughly chopped
100 ml/⅓ cup plain bio yogurt
100 ml/⅓ cup milk of choice
1 heaped tablespoon soya protein powder
   (see page 18)
1 teaspoon lacuma powder (see page 16)
1 teaspoon baobab powder (see page 14)
   or maca powder (see page 16)
½ teaspoon ground cinnamon
granola, for sprinkling

SERVES 2

Put the blackberries, pears, yogurt, milk, soya protein, lacuma, baobab and cinnamon in a blender and blend until smooth. Pour into glasses and spoon the granola on top. Eat with a spoon!

Peach melba smoothie

Inspired by the classic dessert invented by the French chef Auguste Escoffier at the Savoy Hotel in London in the 1893, this peach melba smoothie says 'summer in a glass' to me.

3 small nectarines, pitted
2 large handfuls of fresh or frozen raspberries
150 ml/⅔ cup plain bio yogurt
2 scoops dairy-free vanilla ice cream
bee pollen, for sprinkling (see page 15)

SERVES 2

Put the nectarines, raspberries, yogurt and ice cream in a blender and blend until smooth. Sprinkle with bee pollen just before serving.

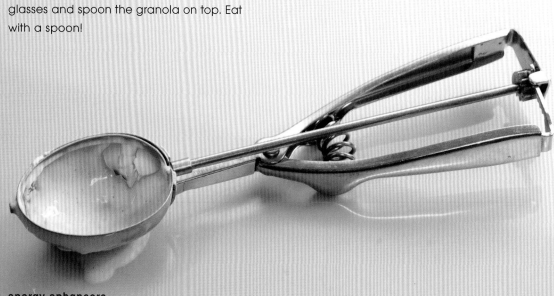

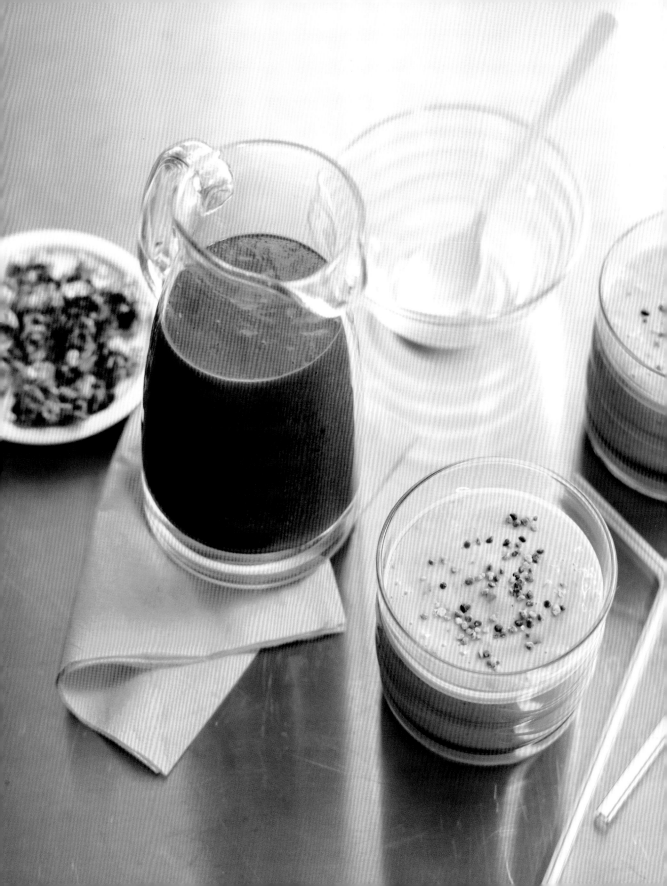

Raspberry and goji restorer

This simple blended drink combines the super-nutrients of raspberries with those of goji berries – a potent combo! Raspberries are particularly rich in brain-boosting B vitamins, which have been found to curb memory loss in later life.

2 tablespoons goji berries

4 large handfuls of raspberries or blueberries

1 large cooked beetroot/beet, chopped

1–2 teaspoons wheatgrass powder (see page 18)

SERVES 2

Soak the goji berries in 3 tablespoons pure or filtered water for 15 minutes until softened, then tip the berries and their soaking liquid into a blender. Add the raspberries, beetroot/beet and wheatgrass powder as well as 250 ml/ 1 cup pure or filtered water, then blend until smooth. If you dislike seeds, strain the juice through a sieve before drinking.

raspberries Alongside giving us an energy boost, the B vitamins found in raspberries have the ability to reduce harmful homocysteine levels, which can hasten the furring up of the arteries. Raspberries can also help to treat menstrual cramps as well as act as a potent detoxifier.

Pea...fect!

Peas may be an unusual addition to a smoothie but the sweet and succulent vegetable is surprisingly good, especially when combined with fresh mint. Frozen petit pois are perfect here, making an incredibly rich and creamy drink, and there's no need to defrost them first.

3 handfuls of frozen petit pois
2 handfuls of mint leaves
2 handfuls of kale, stalks discarded, leaves shredded
300 ml/1¼ cups coconut water (*see page 54*)
½ teaspoon virgin coconut oil
½–1 teaspoon chlorella powder (*see page 15*)

SERVES 2

Put the petit pois, mint, kale, coconut water, coconut oil and chlorella in a blender and blend until smooth. Add extra coconut water if too thick.

peas An energy-giving combination of fibre, protein and carbs, peas also contain an assortment of health-protecting phytonutrients particularly saponins, which have been found to boost the immune system, reduce harmful LDL cholesterol and help to eliminate toxins.

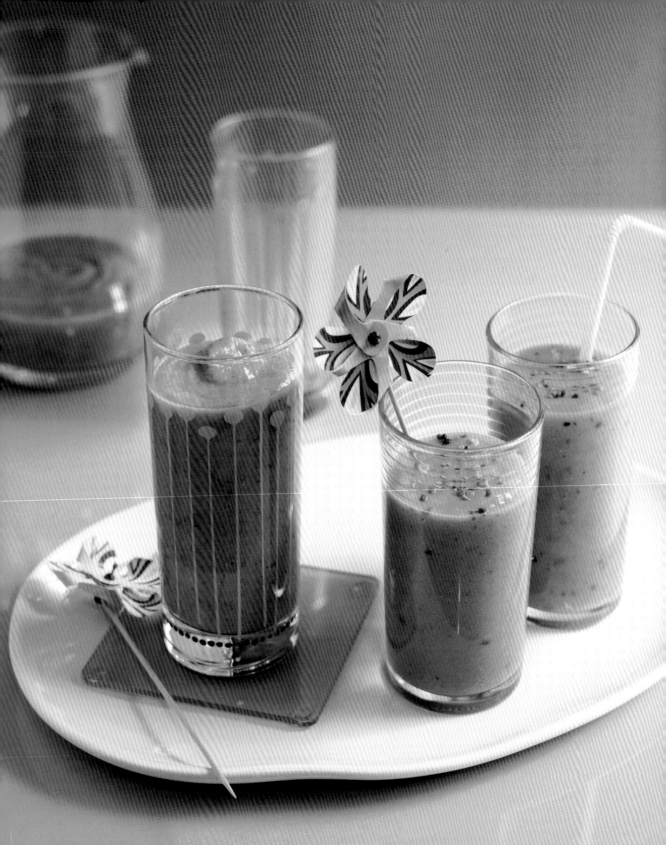

Date and cashew restorer

I made this creamy smoothie after a bout of illness and it was just the thing to give an energy boost when I didn't feel like anything too heavy or solid. Similarly, it would make an energy-giving afternoon snack if you're feeling lacklustre after a hectic day.

10 ready-to-eat dried dates, halved
250 ml/1 cup cashew nut milk *(see page 22)*
4 medium pears, peeled, cored and sliced
1 handful of alfalfa sprouts *(see page 21)*
½ teaspoon vanilla extract
2 teaspoons ground flaxseeds *(see page 16)*
2 teaspoons maca powder *(see page 16)*

SERVES 2

Soak the dates in 5 tablespoons water overnight. The next day, put the cashew nut milk, dates and their soaking liquid into a blender with the pears, alfalfa sprouts, vanilla, flaxseeds and maca powder and blend until smooth and creamy.

cashews Rich in iron, magnesium and selenium as well as phytochemicals, antioxidants and energy-boosting protein, cashews offer us an abundance of nutrients. Their rich copper content is said to improve bone, hair and skin health.

Get your oats

This malty, thick smoothie is rich in vitamins, especially B and C, as well as the minerals iron and potassium. Iron plays a variety of roles in the body and deficiency of the mineral can lead to fatigue, anaemia and poor immunity.

2 large nectarines, pitted and chopped
2 medium bananas, peeled and sliced
200 ml/generous ¾ cup oat milk
½ teaspoon ground cinnamon
1 teaspoon lacuma powder *(see page 16)*
1 teaspoon baobab powder *(see page 14)*
bee pollen *(see page 15)*, for sprinkling

SERVES 2

Put the nectarines, bananas, oat milk, cinnamon, lacuma and baobab into a blender and blend until smooth. Serve sprinkled with bee pollen.

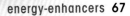

The energiser

Just the thing if you're in need of a caffeine fix! The coffee combined with energy-giving maca, bananas and raw cacao are sure to get you going – just the one will liven you up for the day ahead.

2 teaspoons good-quality coffee granules
250 ml/1 cup almond milk *(see page 22)* or milk
   of choice
75 ml/scant ⅓ cup plain bio yogurt
2 medium bananas, peeled and chopped
½ teaspoon vanilla extract
½ teaspoon ground cinnamon
2 teaspoons maca powder *(see page 16)*
1 teaspoon cacao powder *(see page 15)*
1–2 teaspoons agave syrup (optional)

SERVES 2

Dissolve the coffee in 100 ml/⅓ cup just-boiled water, then allow to cool. Pour the coffee into a blender with the nut milk then add the yogurt, bananas, vanilla, cinnamon, maca and raw cacao and blend until smooth. Taste and, if you like a sweeter smoothie, stir in the agave syrup.

Vanilla shake

Creamy, sustaining and soothing, this shake will pep you up if you're feeling slightly tender after an illness and are in need of a bit of oomph to get you back to speed. Look for good-quality vanilla protein powder, or you could use soya or hemp protein powders instead.

300 ml/1¼ cups coconut drinking milk
100 ml/⅓ cup plain bio yogurt
1 tablespoon vanilla protein powder *(see page 18)*
1 teaspoon vanilla extract
2 small bananas, peeled and chopped
½ teaspoon ground cinnamon
½ teaspoon freshly grated nutmeg
2 teaspoons ground flaxseeds *(see page 16)*
1–2 teaspoons camu camu powder *(see page 15)*

SERVES 2

Put the coconut drinking milk, yogurt, protein powder, vanilla extract, bananas, cinnamon, nutmeg, ground flaxseeds and camu camu powder in a blender and blend until smooth. Add more coconut drinking milk if too thick.

yogurt The 'friendly' bacteria present in live yogurt aid digestion and benefit the internal flora of the gut, particularly valuable after a bout of food poisoning or a course of antibiotics.

coffee Coffee is a doubled-edged sword and can have both bad and good effects on our health. The good news is that it is rich in antioxidants, and is an anti-inflammatory as well as an energy and brain booster, but do drink it in moderation.

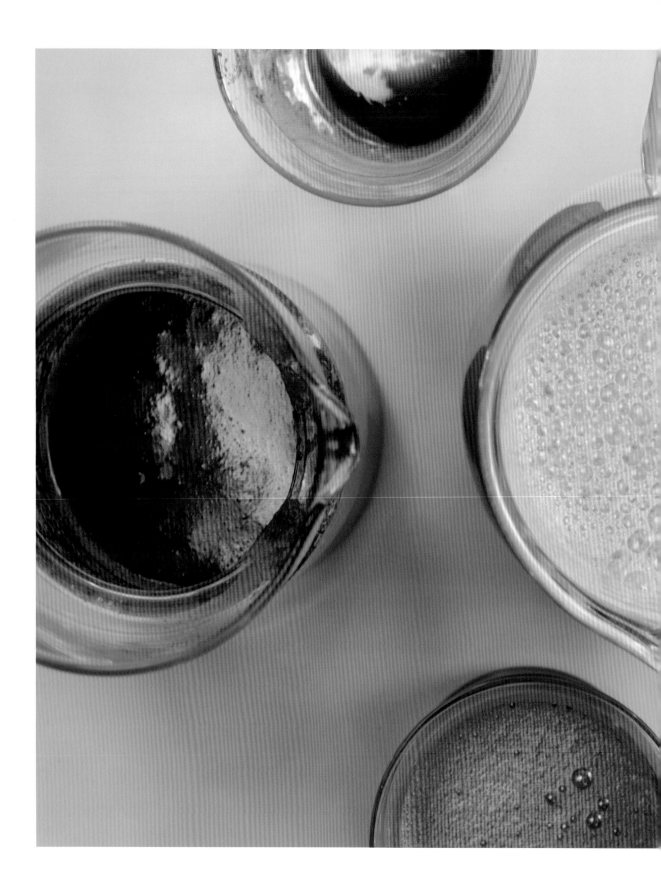

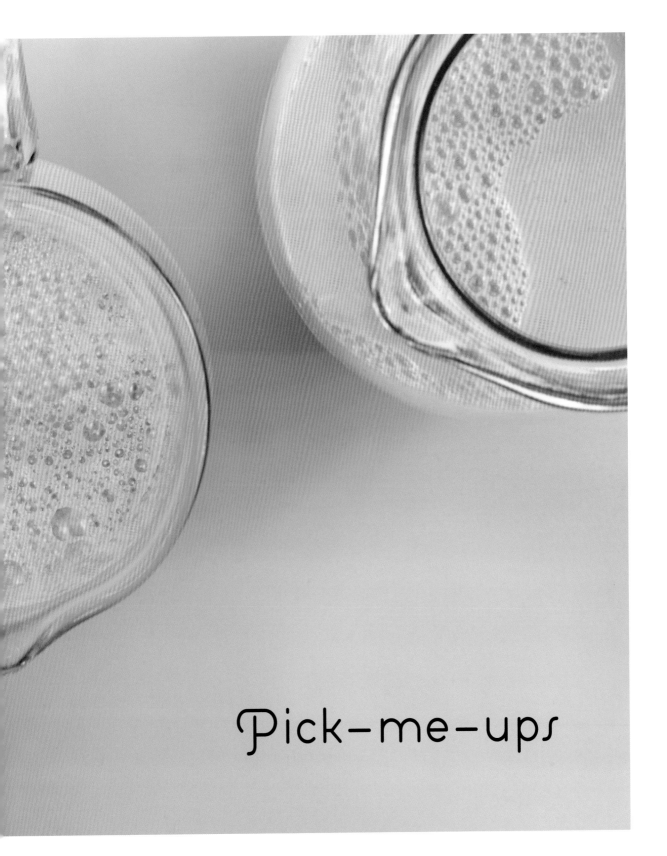

Pick-me-ups

Tangerine dream

Packed with vitamin C, valued for its ability to help boost the immune system and fight infection, this simple, zingy juice looks as good as it tastes. The dried cranberry powder adds an intense burst of flavour – fruit powders come in a range of varieties and you can buy them online.

2 apples, quartered, cored and cut into wedges
4 tangerines or satsumas, peeled and halved
seeds from 2 pomegranates
1 teaspoon dried cranberry powder (*see page 18*)
1 teaspoon açaí berry powder (*see page 14*)
SERVES 2

Juice the apples, tangerines and pomegranates then stir in the cranberry and açaí berry powders.

Pomegranate perfection

Pomegranates are a bit of a fiddle to prepare as you need to remove all the seeds before you start, yet they are well worth it for their colour and flavour. They also produce a surprisingly generous amount of juice despite the high amount of seeds.

1 medium pineapple, peeled, cored and
    cut into long wedges
seeds from 1 large pomegranate
1 teaspoon lemon juice
2 teaspoons camu camu powder (*see page 15*)
SERVES 2

Juice the pineapple and pomegranate then stir in the lemon juice and camu camu.

> **pineapple** benefits the digestive system thanks to the presence of the antibacterial enzyme bromelain. It is also an anti-inflammatory, helping arthritis sufferers, and is an excellent source of vitamin C, manganese and other antioxidants.

cranberry has long been recognised for its ability to curb cystitis and other infections of the urinary tract and, more recently, has been found to reduce levels of bacteria in the bladder and kidneys. It also has anti-inflammatory properties and supports the immune system thanks to the valuable amount of phytonutrients.

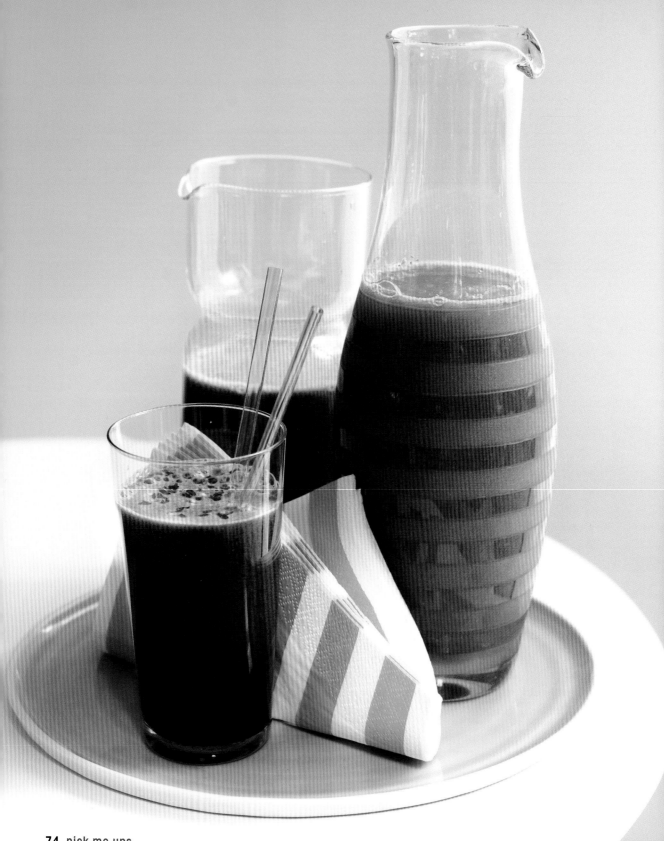

Virgin Mary

Echinacea is traditionally used to fight colds, flu and other infections and works by stimulating the immune system. Make sure you choose ripe tomatoes since that's when they are at their most nutritious.

7 ripe, vine-ripened tomatoes, halved or quartered

4 large carrots, peeled and halved lengthways

2 large handfuls of sliced red cabbage

1 celery stalk, halved crossways

2–3 teaspoons Worcestershire sauce

a few echinacea drops (*see page 18*)

  (*check the recommended dosage on the bottle*)

chopped fresh chilli/chile or chilli/red pepper flakes,

  for sprinkling (*optional*)

SERVES 2

Juice the tomatoes, carrots, red cabbage and celery then stir in the Worcestershire sauce and echinacea drops. Serve sprinkled with chilli/chile.

Orange zing

The vibrant, sunset orange colour of this juice is enough to pick me up after a long, stressful day. Super rich in vitamin C, it makes an effective digestive aid and immune system booster.

2 large oranges, peeled and split into wedges

4 good handfuls of skinned and deseeded

  watermelon

juice of 2 large limes

2 teaspoons baobab powder (*see page 14*)

½ teaspoon finely grated orange zest

SERVES 2

Juice the oranges and watermelon then stir in the lime juice and baobab. Sprinkle with a little orange zest before drinking.

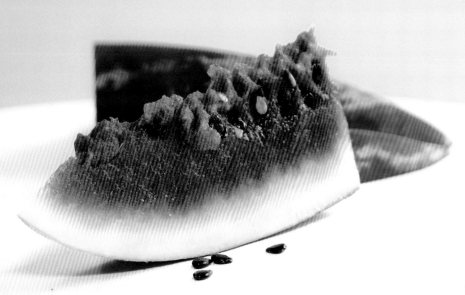

Sweet as...

Nurturing and sustaining, this juice provides a valuable cocktail of nutrients, protein and carbohydrates – just what you need to get you back to good health after a bout of illness. The Peruvian fruit camu camu gives us impressive levels of immune-boosting vitamin C.

1 medium sweet potato, peeled and cut into long wedges

2 large Chinese leaves, each halved and rolled up

1 medium red (bell) pepper, deseeded and cut into long wedges

2-cm/¾-inch piece fresh root ginger, peeled

2 tablespoons pumpkin seeds

1–2 teaspoons wheatgrass powder (*see page 18*) or camu camu extract powder (*see page 15*)

¼ teaspoon bee pollen

SERVES 2

Juice the sweet potato, Chinese leaves, red (bell) pepper, ginger and pumpkin seeds, adding a splash of pure or filtered water if your machine struggles with the seeds. Stir in the wheatgrass powder or camu camu powder and sprinkle with bee pollen.

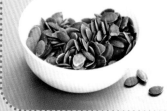

pumpkin seeds For their size, pumpkin seeds pack a powerful punch. Most notable is their iron content: a 50 g/2 oz. serving provides almost three-quarters of our daily requirement.

Apple a day

Severe stress can affect the whole body and the way it functions, including the digestive system. At times like this, it's often easier on the body to consume nutrients in liquid form, rather than use precious energy to digest solids. This juice provides a good range of nutrients, including the rejuvenating properties of spirulina.

4 carrots, peeled and halved lengthways

1 apple, quartered, cored and cut into wedges

3 handfuls of seedless white grapes

2 handfuls of sliced red cabbage

1 teaspoon lemon juice

1–2 teaspoons spirulina (see page 18)

SERVES 2

Juice the carrots, apple, grapes and cabbage then stir in the lemon juice and spirulina.

lemon The immune-boosting properties of vitamin C are well documented and are found in bountiful amounts in lemons. While unlikely to prevent colds and flu, the nutrient certainly lessens their severity and the length of illness. Vitamin C also increases the body's ability to absorb iron from food.

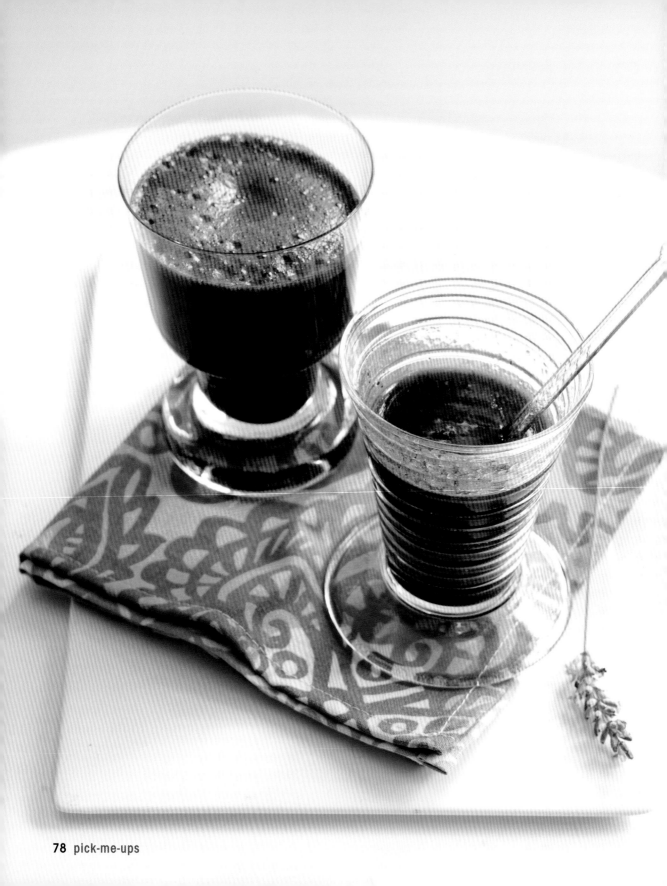

Reishi healing

Reishi mushrooms, used here in a powdered form, help to regulate the immune system as well as improve the functioning of the organs in the body – and that's just for starters. They are most effective when eaten in conjunction with a source of vitamin C, at the beginning of the day and on an empty stomach.

1 medium sweet potato, peeled and cut into
   long wedges
1 small raw beetroot/beet, peeled and
   cut into wedges
2 apples, quartered, cored and cut into wedges
2 teaspoons lemon juice
2 teaspoons reishi mushroom powder (*see page 17*)

SERVES 2

Juice the sweet potato, beetroot/beet and apples, then stir in the lemon juice and reishi powder.

Summer nectar

Rich and berry red, a gulp of this juice will take you back to the summer. Lavender is known for its calmative properties, so it's great taken when you're feeling stressed. It also treats gastrointestinal problems and can be an effective pain relief. Check the lavender is edible and hasn't been sprayed with pesticides before use.

2 lavender flowers, stem removed
4 peaches, pitted
4 handfuls of raspberries
3 handfuls of pitted frozen dark cherries, defrosted
2 teaspoons açaí berry powder (*see page 14*)

SERVES 2

Steep the lavender in 100 ml/⅓ cup just-boiled water and leave to infuse for 1 hour. Just before serving, juice the peaches, raspberries and cherries. Strain the lavender water, discard the flowers and stir the soaking water into the juice with the açaí berry powder until combined.

peaches Called the 'longevity' fruit in traditional Chinese medicine, the peach is an excellent source of the antioxidants beta carotene and vitamin C as well as the mineral potassium. A shortage of potassium has been linked to an increased risk of heart disease along with anxiety, fatigue, poor memory and muscle weakness.

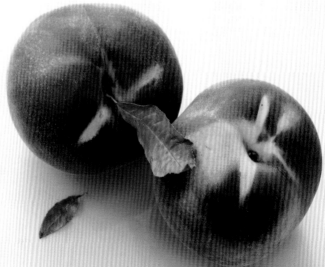

Sporty reviver

Knock this back after a session at the gym to perk up low energy levels. It's not just vitamin C that's prevalent in this juice, but also a wide range of immune-protective flavonoids.

6 carrots, peeled and halved lengthways

2 kiwis, peeled and halved

4 small handfuls of spinach

1 red grapefruit, peeled and split into segments

1 teaspoon lacuma powder *(see page 16)*

1–2 teaspoons powdered greens *(see page 17)*

SERVES 2

Juice the carrots, kiwi, spinach and grapefruit, then stir in the lacuma and powdered greens.

Cold comfort

Warm, spicy and restorative – just the thing if you're run down with a cold or flu and need a pick-me-up.

4 cloves

½ cinnamon stick

2 apples, peeled, cored and chopped

2 large handfuls of blackcurrants

1 teaspoon manuka honey *(see page 16)*

2 teaspoons ginger cordial

SERVES 2

Put the cloves and cinnamon stick in 400 ml/ 1⅔ cups just-boiled water and allow to infuse for 1 hour. Remove the cloves and cinnamon stick and pour the water into a blender, then add the apples, blackcurrants, honey and ginger cordial and blend until smooth.

blackcurrants In natural medicine, blackcurrants are prescribed to settle an upset stomach, but there's no ignoring their impressive vitamin C content. The vitamin is especially good for reducing the symptoms of a cold.

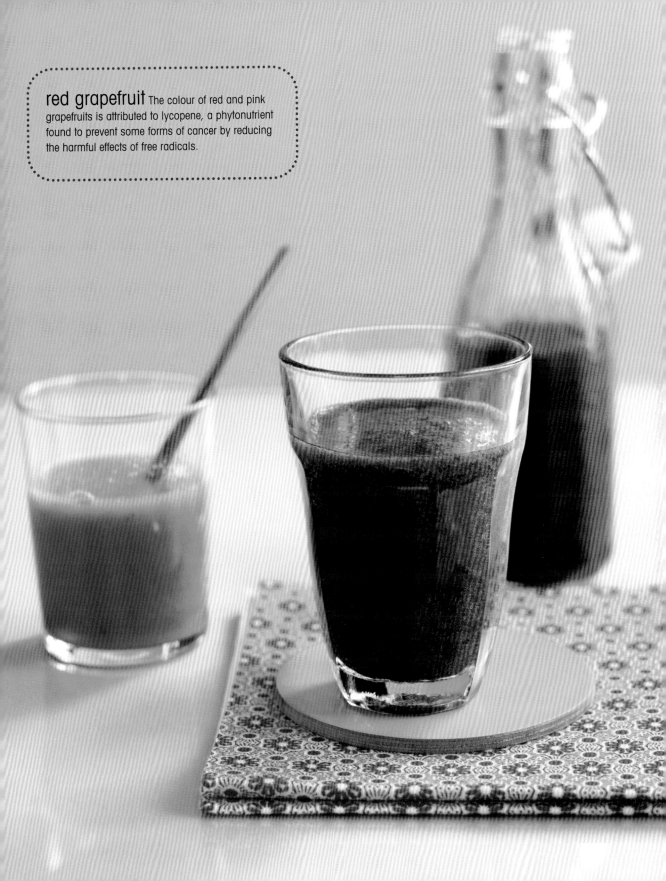

red grapefruit The colour of red and pink grapefruits is attributed to lycopene, a phytonutrient found to prevent some forms of cancer by reducing the harmful effects of free radicals.

Citrus sherbert

I love the stunning deep orange colour of this blended juice; it looks almost as good as it tastes and is a true pick-me-up when you're feeling a bit groggy! This would also make a good thirst-quenching long drink topped up with sparkling mineral water.

6 large handfuls of chopped watermelon, deseeded
4 clementines, peeled and quartered
juice of 1 lime
2 teaspoons baobab powder (*see page 14*)
SERVES 2

Put the watermelon, clementines, lime juice and baobab powder in a blender and blend until smooth.

watermelon may have a high water content and be low in calories, but it is an excellent source of lycopene, a carotenoid that is important for eye and bone health; do make sure it is ripe for the highest nutritional status. The seeds also provide useful amounts of iron and zinc so if you're not adverse to a bit of crunch, do reserve a few to add to the fruit before blending.

Mango chai

Spices add a wonderful flavour boost and they're good for you too, especially benefitting the digestive system. The blend of mango, carrot, spices and white tea is restorative and packed with antioxidants that have been found to protect cells from cancer-causing substances.

cardamom This fragrant spice calms indigestion and has been found to relieve colds and coughs.

1 white tea bag
1 cinnamon stick
3 cardamom pods, split
1 medium mango, peeled, pitted and cubed
1 medium carrot, peeled and grated
1-cm/½-inch piece fresh root ginger, peeled
   and chopped
½ teaspoon ground turmeric
2 probiotic powder (*see page 18*)
   (*check the recommended dosage on the bottle*)
few drops echinacea (*see page 18*)
   (*check the recommended dosage on the bottle*)
SERVES 2

Put the white tea bag in a cup of 300 ml/
1¼ cups just-boiled water. Add the cinnamon stick and cardamom and allow to steep for 5 minutes, then remove the bag and allow the tea to cool and infuse. When cool, remove the spices and pour the tea into a blender. Add the mango, carrot, ginger, turmeric and probiotic powder and blend until smooth. Pour into glasses and stir in the echinacea.

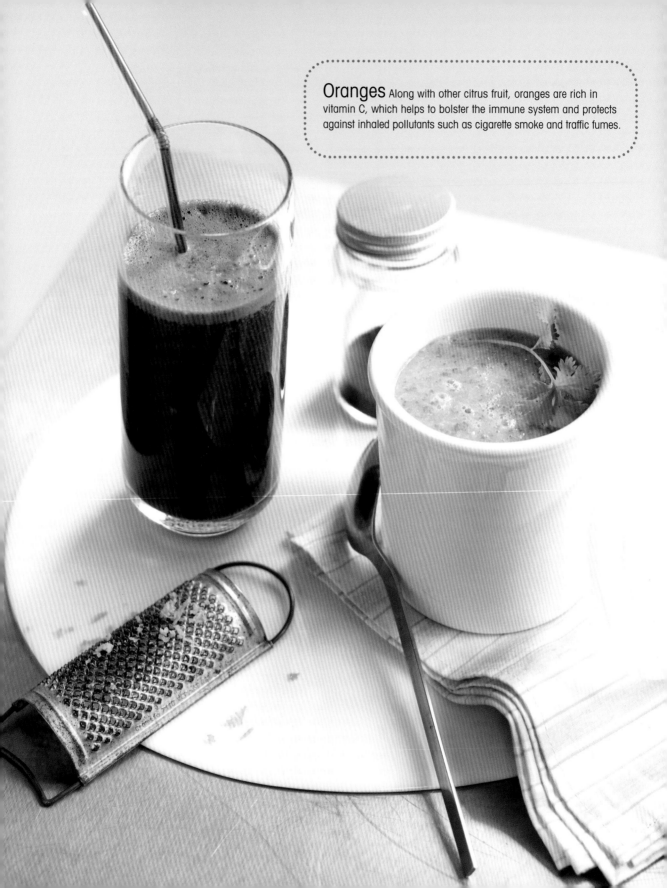

Oranges Along with other citrus fruit, oranges are rich in vitamin C, which helps to bolster the immune system and protects against inhaled pollutants such as cigarette smoke and traffic fumes.

Chocolate–orange shake

Rich, dark and indulgent, this is the perfect partnership of raw cacao and fresh orange. Aloe vera juice is highly regarded for its plentiful health-giving properties, but do look for a high-potency, whole-leaf brand.

juice of 3 oranges
10 ready-to-eat dried dates, sliced
2 small handfuls of blanched almonds
2 teaspoons raw cacao powder (*see page 15*)
2 teaspoons açaí berry powder (*see page 14*)
aloe vera juice (*see page 14*)
   (*check the recommended dosage on the bottle*)
½ teaspoon finely grated orange zest

SERVES 2

Put the orange juice, almonds, raw cacao powder, açaí berry powder and aloe vera juice in a blender and blend until almost smooth – the nuts may give a slight texture to the shake, but you can strain it if you like. Serve sprinkled with orange zest.

Avocado smoopie

A cross between a smoothie and soup, this makes a nutritious snack or light lunch. It's a delicious, rejuvenating combination of creamy avocado, fresh coriander/cilantro, delicate cucumber with just a hint of chilli/chile.

1 medium avocado, stoned, peeled and chopped
½ cucumber, deseeded and sliced
2 spring onions/scallions, chopped
2 tablespoons chopped coriander/cilantro leaves
1 green chilli/chile, deseeded and sliced
250 ml/1 cup coconut water (*see page 54*)
splash of Tabasco sauce
juice of 1 lime
5 ice cubes
1–2 teaspoons spirulina powder (*see page 18*)

SERVES 2

Put the avocado, cucumber, spring onions/scallions, coriander/cilantro, green chilli/chile, coconut water, Tabasco, lime juice, ice cubes and spirulina in a blender and blend until smooth and creamy.

fresh coriander/cilantro
This fresh herb is an effective digestive, easing stomach pains, indigestion and nausea. It is also believed to be a tonic for the heart.

Cherry aid

*This is the perfect midday booster –
something sweet to follow lunch and with
battery-fuelling properties. It's rich in iron,
vitamin C, carotenoids and anthocyanidins,
which all have protective and regenerative
properties.*

3 good handfuls of frozen, pitted dark cherries
2 handfuls of baby spinach leaves
375 ml/1½ cups almond milk *(see page 22)*
2 tablespoons rolled oats
½ teaspoon vanilla extract
2 teaspoons raw cacao powder *(see page 15)*
½ teaspoon ground cinnamon, plus extra for sprinkling
2 teaspoons açaí berry powder *(see page 14)*

SERVES 2

Put the cherries, spinach, almond milk, oats,
vanilla, raw cacao, cinnamon and açaí berry
powder in a blender and blend until smooth.

Avocado baby

*This definitely tastes a lot better than it looks,
but don't be put off as you don't want to
miss its fruity, chocolatey taste and thick,
creamy consistency. What's more, it has
many restorative properties and helps to
give energy levels a real boost.*

½ medium avocado, peeled and sliced
1 small mango, peeled, pitted and chopped
juice of 3 oranges
2 teaspoons soya protein powder *(see page 18)*
½ teaspoon ground nutmeg
1–2 teaspoons barleygrass powder *(see page 14)*
2 teaspoons raw cacao powder *(see page 15)*

SERVES 2

Put the avocado, mango, orange juice, protein
powder, nutmeg, barleygrass and raw cacao
powder in a blender and blend until smooth.

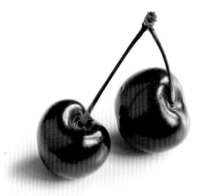

cherries Cleansing and rejuvenating, cherries
contain a potent anti-inflammatory used to treat the
symptoms of gout and arthritis as well as encouraging
the elimination of toxins from the kidneys.

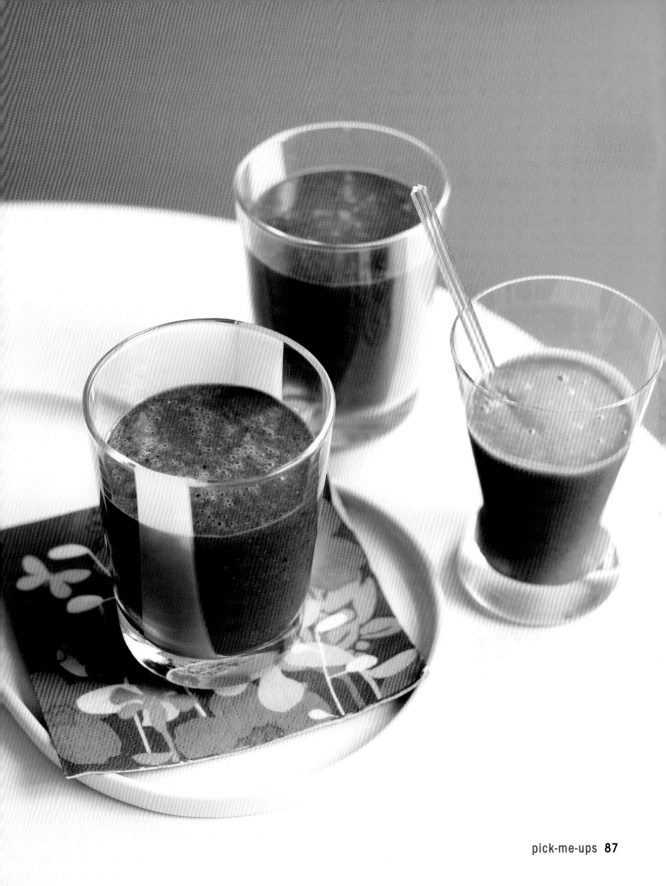

fruit powders

Dried fruit powders make
a convenient alternative to
their fresh equivalent and
are a simple way to add a
nutritious flavour boost to
juices and smoothies.

Brain booster

Just a single Brazil nut a day provides the recommended amount of the mineral selenium, which is excellent for the brain and a great mood enhancer.

1 small handful of goji berries
200 ml/generous ¾ cup plain bio yogurt
150 ml/⅔ cup coconut drinking milk
3 Brazil nuts
1 tablespoon hemp protein powder (*see page 18*)
2 handfuls of blueberries
1 teaspoon blackcurrant powder (*see page 18*)
1 teaspoon camu camu powder (*see page 15*)

SERVES 2

Soak the goji berries in 4 tablespoons warm water for 30 minutes until softened. Put the goji, soaking water, yogurt, coconut drinking milk, Brazil nuts, hemp protein powder, blueberries, blackcurrant powder and camu camu powder in a blender and blend until smooth.

Mint choc chip

The classic combination of mint and chocolate comes together in this creamy, satisfying smoothie – just the thing if you need a pick-me-up after an illness or a particularly stressful time.

3 medium bananas, peeled and chopped
2 scoops dairy-free vanilla ice cream
300 ml/1¼ cups dairy-free milk
1 teaspoon raw cacao powder (*see page 15*)
½ teaspoon vanilla extract
2 teaspoons maca powder (*see page 16*)
1 teaspoon chopped fresh mint
raw cacao nibs, for sprinkling (*see page 15*)

SERVES 2

Put the bananas, dairy-free ice cream, dairy-free milk, raw cacao powder, vanilla extract and maca powder in a blender and blend until smooth and creamy. Stir in the mint and sprinkle the cacao nibs over the top.

raw cacao is the unprocessed seed of the cocoa tree. It comes in various forms including a powder, nibs or butter. It's a good source of iron, dietary fibre, magnesium, antioxidants and essential fatty acids. It also contains the amino acid tryptophan said to enhance relaxation and promote better sleep as well as theobromine, a mild stimulant that can help lift depression.

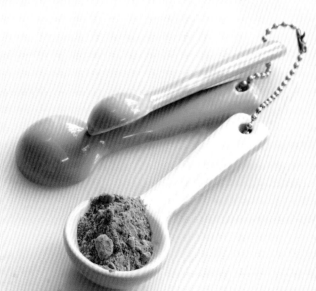

Tropical spice

Rich and nurturing, this smoothie is a delicious combination of tropical fruit and spices. When choosing a pineapple, tug one of the leaves on top and if it comes away easily, it is ripe and ready to eat.

½ large pineapple, peeled, cored and chopped
1 banana, peeled and chopped
200 ml/generous ¾ cup plain bio yogurt
100 ml/⅓ cup coconut drinking milk
½ teaspoon ground ginger
1 teaspoon manuka honey (*see page 16*)
1 teaspoon lime juice
seeds from 3 cardamom pods, ground
½ teaspoon finely grated lime zest
ice, to serve (optional)

SERVES 2

Put the pineapple, banana, yogurt, coconut drinking milk, ginger, honey and lime juice in blender and blend until smooth and creamy. Stir in the ground cardamom and pour into glasses. Add a few ice cubes, if you like, and sprinkle with the lime zest.

Breakfast shake

Blueberries, as well as being excellent for the health of the eyes, are effective in treating urinary tract infections and improving poor circulation, while raspberries help to remove toxins. They work in tandem to repair and revitalise the body.

2 handfuls of blueberries
2 handfuls of frozen or fresh raspberries
juice of 2 large oranges
2 teaspoons manuka honey (*see page 16*)
2 tablespoons jumbo oats
2 teaspoons açaí berry powder (*see page 14*)

SERVES 2

Put the blueberries, raspberries, orange juice, honey, oats and açaí berry powder in a blender and blend until smooth.

jumbo oats High in fibre, oats also contain protease inhibitors, a combination that has been found to reduce the incidence of certain cancers. Oats provide B vitamins, vitamin E, iron, magnesium, calcium and potassium, too.

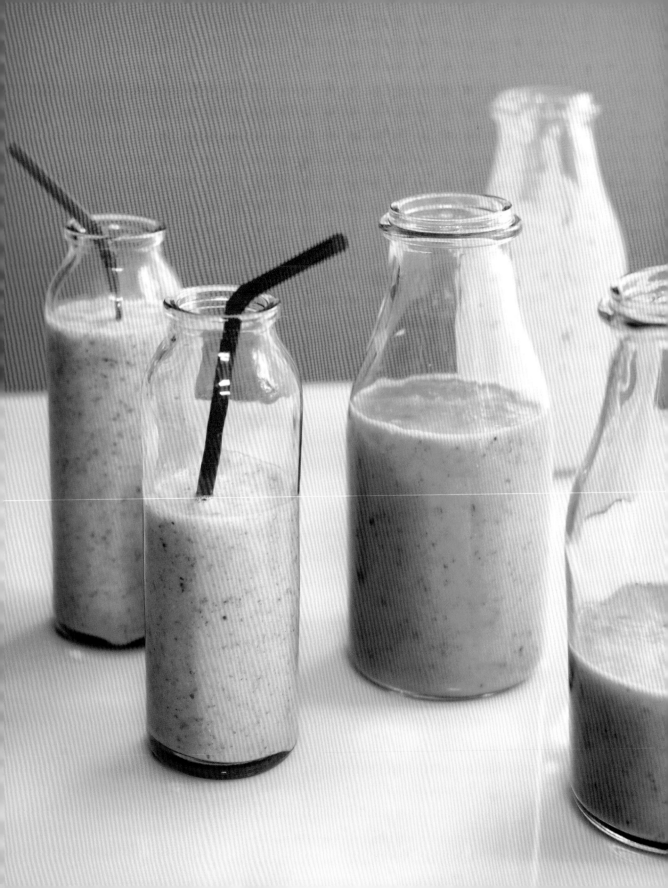

Virgin piña colada

There's no need to soak the dates in this creamy, coconutty drink if they're nice and soft, but if on the dry side, allow to soak in water for 30 minutes. This is just the thing if you feel you need a protein-packed energy boost.

2 tablespoons sunflower seeds
250 ml/1 cup coconut drinking milk
½ small pineapple, peeled, cored and chopped
2 ready-to-eat dried dates, halved
1 tablespoon light tahini paste
2 teaspoons baobab powder (*see page 14*)
2 teaspoons ground flaxseeds (*see page 16*)
ice, to serve (*optional*)

SERVES 2

Soak the sunflower seeds in 2 tablespoons pure or filtered water for 15 minutes. Put the coconut drinking milk, pineapple, dates, tahini paste, baobab powder, flaxseeds and the sunflower seeds with their soaking water in a blender and blend until smooth and creamy. Serve with ice, if you like.

Strawberry and vanilla booster

The classic combinations are the best and you can't beat the partnership of strawberries and vanilla. This goes one better with the inclusion of pear and banana for a real fruit explosion.

3 good handfuls of strawberries, hulled
1 banana, peeled and sliced
2 pears, peeled, cored and chopped
300 ml/1¼ cups oat milk
50 ml/3½ tablespoons natural bio yogurt
½ teaspoon mixed spice
½ teaspoon vanilla extract
2 teaspoons maca powder (*see page 16*)

SERVES 2

Put the strawberries, banana, pears, oat milk, yogurt, mixed spice, vanilla extract and maca powder in a blender and blend until smooth.

sunflower seeds Recognized for their restorative qualities in natural medicine, sunflower seeds give us linoleic acid, otherwise known as omega-6 fats, which have been found to reduce harmful LDL cholesterol in the body.

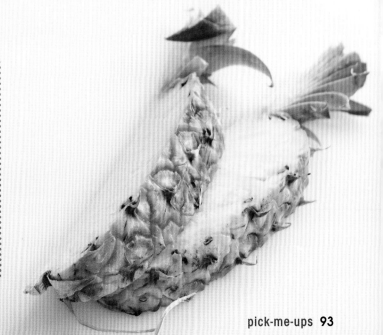

Merry cherry

I've used frozen cherries for this smoothie as they come ready-pitted, saving the hassle of removing the stones – and there's no need to defrost them first. Purple-skinned plums don't just add a great colour and flavour, they are also rich in antioxidants, good for digestion and the blood – make sure they're ripe though.

1 star anise
2 tablespoons goji berries
175 ml/¾ cup coconut water (*see page 54*)
2 large handfuls of pitted frozen dark cherries
4 purple plums, halved and pitted
½ teaspoon ground cinnamon
50 ml/3½ tablespoons natural bio yogurt
1 tablespoon flaked quinoa

SERVES 2

Soak the star anise and goji berries in 50 ml/ 3½ tablespoons hot water for 1 hour. Remove the star anise and tip the goji and the soaking water into a blender with the coconut water, cherries, plums, ground cinnamon, yogurt and quinoa, then blend until smooth and creamy.

> **plums** In addition to relieving constipation thanks to their high fibre content, plums are a good source of vitamin C, beta carotene and vitamin K. Eating extra vitamin C around the cold or flu season is a sensible idea.

Full of passion

The passion fruit gives a wonderful tropical flavour to this reviving blend, which is one of my favourites when in need of a pick-me-up and instant energy boost.

3 passion fruit, halved and fruit scooped out
4 handfuls of strawberries, hulled
juice of 1 pink grapefruit
10 basil leaves
small handful of mint leaves
1–2 teaspoons maca powder (*see page 16*)
1 teaspoon baobab powder (*see page 14*)

SERVES 2

Put the passion fruit flesh, strawberries, grapefruit juice, basil, mint, maca and baobab powder in a blender and blend until smooth.

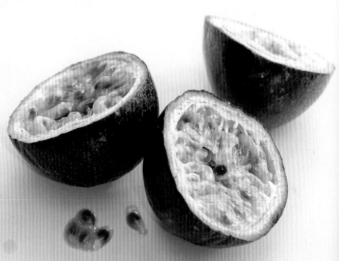

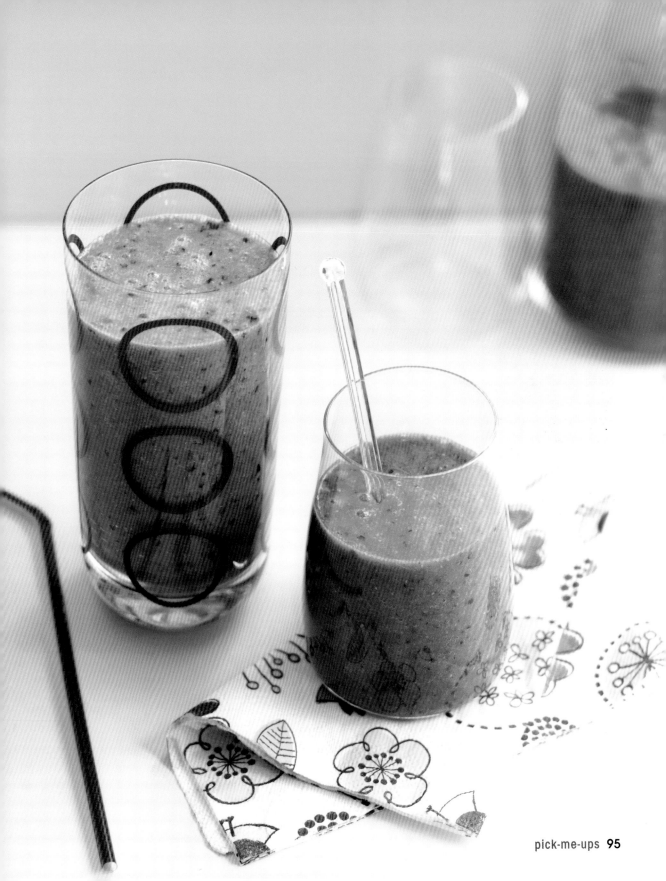

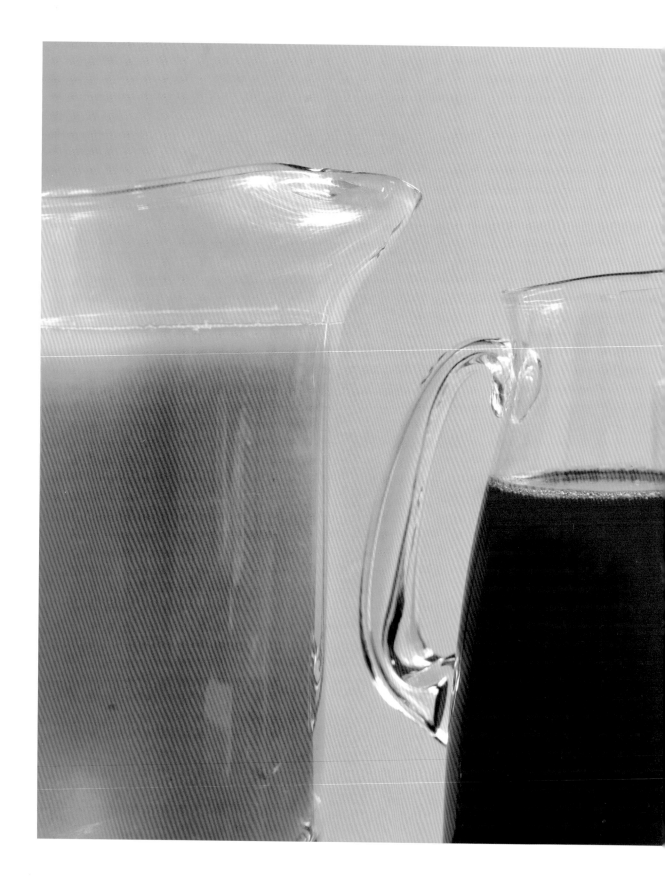

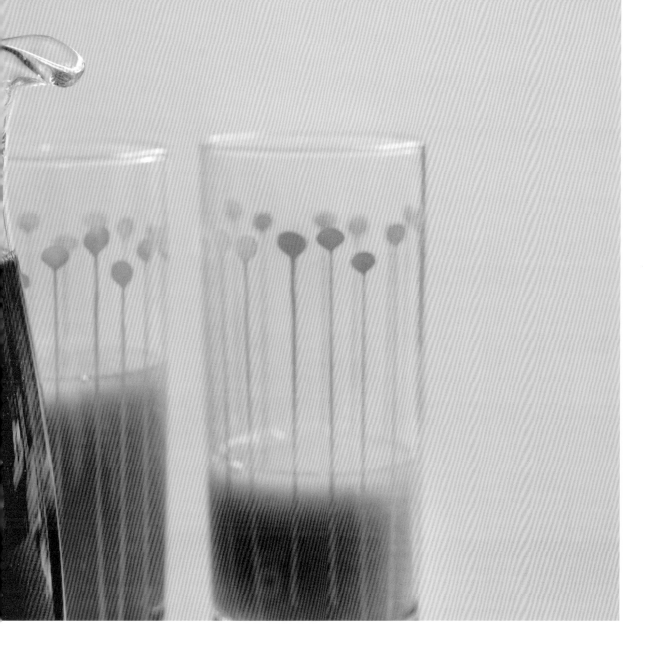

Weight-loss aids

Berry good

The pears add a hint of sweetness to this mildly aniseedy juice. It makes a good energy-boosting drink mid-afternoon if you need something to help keep you going through to dinnertime.

2 medium carrots, peeled and halved lengthways
1 Little Gem lettuce, leaves separated
½ medium fennel bulb, cut into long wedges
1 small handful of flat-leaf parsley
2 pears, quartered and cored
1 teaspoon lemon juice
2 teaspoons açaí berry powder (*see page 14*)

SERVES 2

Juice the carrots, lettuce, fennel, parsley and pears. Stir in the lemon juice and açaí berries.

lettuce is nutritionally most potent when eaten raw. Despite being 90 per cent water, it contains useful amounts of vitamins and minerals, particularly iron, folates, vitamins A and C. The outer, darker leaves tend to be more nutrient dense than the paler inner leaves so it's best to juice the whole thing and drink straightaway before it discolours.

Super-duper juice

I would say this super green juice falls into the 'good for you' category, rather than the super tasty – not that it's offensive, just a bit 'green'! It's worth having a go at growing your own sprouted seeds and beans and it is very easy to do; turn to page 21 for full instructions.

3 apples, quartered, cored and cut into wedges
3 handfuls of spinach
1 handful of broccoli sprouts
2 handfuls of seedless white grapes
2 teaspoons lime juice
1–2 teaspoons barleygrass powder (*see page 14*)
¼ teaspoon chia seeds (*see page 15*)

SERVES 2

Juice the apples, spinach, broccoli sprouts and grapes. Stir in the lime juice, barleygrass and chia seeds.

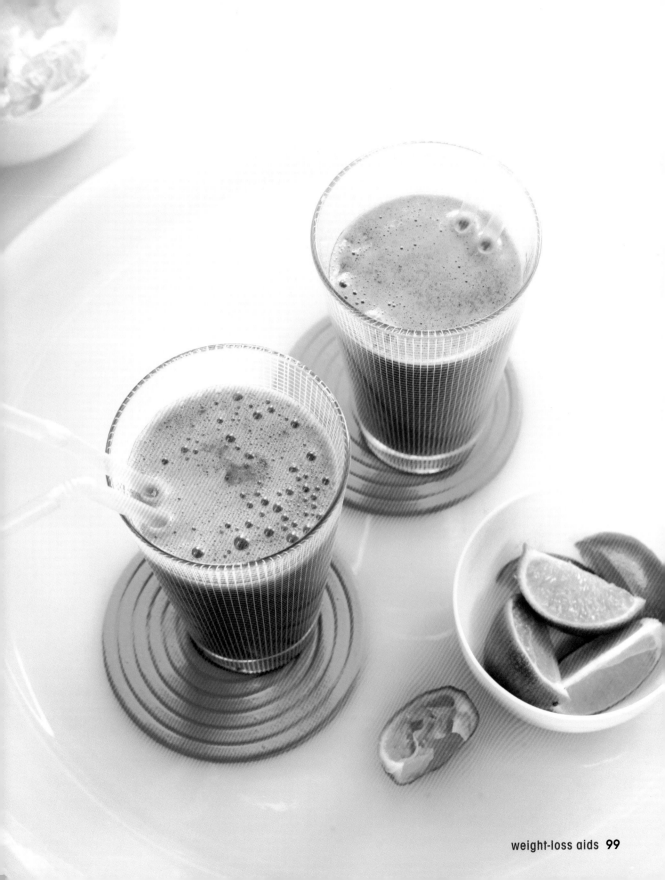

Gazpacho smoopie

This is a cross between a juice or smoothie and a soup, otherwise known as a 'smoopie'. It's delicious served on ice for a summery light lunch. The tomatoes are very juicy so it's a good idea to put them through the juicer more than once to extract every last drop.

2 large, vine-ripened beefsteak tomatoes,
   cut into wedges
2 medium carrots, peeled and halved lengthways
1 small red (bell) pepper, deseeded and cut into
   long wedges
1 stick celery, cut in half
½ cucumber, quartered lengthways
3 medium radishes, halved
½ teaspoon flaxseed oil
few drops Tabasco sauce
juice of ½ lemon
small clove garlic, minced
1–2 teaspoons barleygrass powder *(see page 14)*
basil leaves, chopped, for sprinkling
ice, to serve (optional)

SERVES 2

Juice the tomatoes, carrots, red (bell) pepper, celery, cucumber, radishes and stir in the flaxseed oil, Tabasco, lemon juice, garlic and barleygrass. Sprinkle with basil and add ice cubes, if you like.

(You could also blend this juice; it will have a thicker consistency so you may need to add some pure or filtered water.)

Tomato turbo

Make sure the tomatoes are ripened on the vine and at room temperature for the best flavour. The pulp was very juicy when I made this so I put it through the juicer three times to extract the maximum amount of liquid; you could also press it through a sieve.

2 large, vine-ripened beefsteak tomatoes,
   cut into wedges
1 medium cucumber, quartered lengthways
½ small fennel bulb, cut into long wedges
juice of ½ lemon
1–2 teaspoons wheatgrass powder *(see page 18)*

SERVES 2

Juice the tomatoes, cucumber and fennel then stir in the lemon juice and wheatgrass powder.

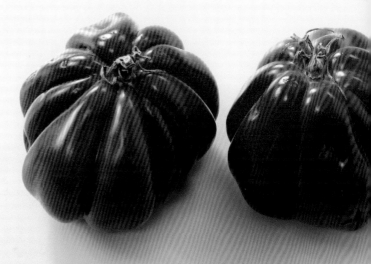

Magic mushrooms

In Chinese medicine, reishi is recommended for regulating and normalizing the function of the main organs of the body. Additionally, it's an adaptogen so helps to maintain and restore overall balance.

3 apples, cored and cut into wedges
1 handful of curly kale
2 medium carrots, peeled and halved lengthways
1 small celery stick
juice of ½ small lemon
2 teaspoons reishi mushroom powder (*see page 17*)

SERVES 2

Juice the apples, kale, carrots and celery, then stir in the lemon juice and reishi powder.

Citrus hit

Sweet potatoes lend a slightly sweet creaminess to this juice in contrast to the citrus zing of the oranges and grapefruit. Grapefruit's reputed fat-burning properties have been attributed to its ability to cause a drop in insulin levels, which in turn curbs the appetite.

1 small sweet potato, peeled and cut into long wedges
2 oranges, peeled and separated into segments
1 pink grapefruit, peeled and separated into segments
¼ fennel bulb, cut into long wedges
1–2 teaspoons camu camu powder (*see page 15*)
1 teaspoon chopped mint leaves

SERVES 2

Juice the sweet potato, oranges, grapefruit and fennel, then stir in the camu camu and chopped mint.

orange Recent research shows it's preferable to get your daily vitamin C intake from natural sources, such as a glass of orange juice, rather than in supplement form. The latter has been found to not provide the same protective qualities.

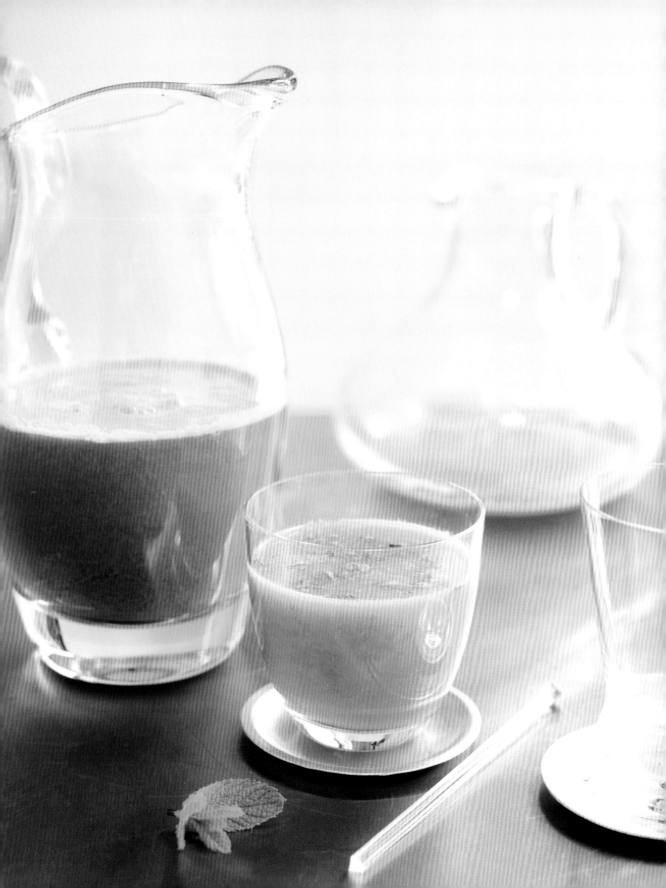

Pepper pot

Chillies/chiles have a stimulating effect, helping to boost the circulation and encourage the release of feel-good chemicals known as endorphins – just the thing if you're struggling to keep up momentum on a weight-loss plan!

Juice the red (bell) peppers, carrots, celery and ginger, then stir in the chilli/chile and spirulina.

2 red (bell) peppers, deseeded cut into long wedges
4 carrots, peeled and halved lengthways
1 celery stick, halved crossways
2.5-cm/1-inch piece fresh root ginger, peeled and halved
½ medium red chilli/chile, deseeded and finely chopped
1–2 teaspoons spirulina powder (see page 18)

SERVES 2

red (bell) pepper Research has shown that red (bell) peppers can increase metabolism through thermogenic action, the process in which the body increases temperature or energy output. Fat is then burned as energy to support the increase in metabolism.

Green for go

Melon and ginger have always been great partners and this refreshing, long drink, topped up with sparkling mineral water is no exception; it's perfect for sipping, helping to curb the appetite and keep you hydrated.

½ medium cucumber, quartered lengthways

¼ large honeydew melon, peeled, deseeded and sliced

2 kiwi fruit, peeled and quartered

1-cm/⅜-inch piece fresh root ginger, unpeeled

juice of ½ lime juice

100 ml/⅓ cup sparkling mineral water

¼ teaspoon chia seeds (*see page 15*)

SERVES 2

Juice the cucumber, melon, kiwi and ginger then stir in the lime juice and sparkling water. Sprinkle the chia seeds over before serving.

kiwi The kiwi's slightly dowdy, fuzzy brown skin hides a vibrant green fruit studded with tiny black seeds. It's packed with vitamin C and is a good source of potassium and fibre.

himalayan pink sea salt

Considered superior to everyday table salt, this pretty pale pink pure crystal salt is rich in minerals in a readily absorbable form. It is also said to help control and regulate water levels in the body, curbing bloating due to water retention.

Aniseed twist

Sweet potatoes are extraordinarily good juiced, producing a vibrant orange, almost creamy drink. They also help regulate blood sugar levels, so keep you sustained for longer and reduce the temptation to snack, while the coconut water keeps you hydrated.

1 large sweet potato, peeled and cut into long chunks
2 carrots, peeled and halved lengthways
½ small fennel bulb, cut into long wedges
300 ml/1¼ cups coconut water
fennel seeds, for sprinkling

SERVES 2

Juice the sweet potato, carrots and fennel bulb. Stir in the coconut water and serve sprinkled with fennel seeds.

> **fennel** Excellent for digestion, fennel has a calming, toning effect on the stomach and is a diuretic. It is also low in calories.

Cucumber cooler

Proper hydration is important on a weight-loss diet. Cucumbers have a high water content so are hydrating as well naturally low in calories, and make a refreshing, summery drink. The pretty pale pink Himalayan sea salt is especially high in minerals and helps to regulate water levels within the body.

1 small cucumber, deseeded and cut into wedges
4 vine-ripened tomatoes, deseeded and cut
   into wedges
1 celery stick, sliced
¼ fennel bulb, cut into long wedges
1 medium red chilli/chile, deseeded and sliced
pinch of Himalayan pink sea salt (optional)
1–2 teaspoons barleygrass powder (*see page 14*)
4 ice cubes
2 teaspoons chopped basil leaves

SERVES 2

Put the cucumber, tomatoes, celery, fennel, chilli/chile, Himalayan pink sea salt, barleygrass and ice cubes in a blender with 100 ml/⅓ cup pure or filtered water and blend until smooth. Sprinkle with the basil before serving.

Sunset glow

With its wonderful colour of a setting sun, this blended juice could make a delicious dessert to follow an evening meal if you're looking for something that is not only sweet but also good for you.

6 unsulphured dried apricots
juice of 3 large oranges
1 large carrot, coarsely grated
juice of 1 small lemon
2 teaspoons açaí berry powder *(see page 14)*

SERVES 2

Soak the apricots in 100 ml/⅓ cup of pure or filtered water for 30 minutes (or overnight if making the juice the next morning). Put the apricots, soaking water, orange juice, carrot, lemon juice and açaí berry powder in a blender and blend until smooth.

Orchard harvest

Intensely fruity, filling and packed with immune-boosting vitamin C. For the best flavour make sure you use fruit that is ripe and in season. You can use shop-bought apple juice but make sure it's a good-quality cloudy juice and not one from made from a concentrate.

2 large handfuls of fresh or frozen blackberries
2 ripe pears, peeled, cored and chopped
2 ripe purple plums, pitted and chopped
200 ml/generous ¾ cup fresh apple juice
   (not from concentrate) or 2 apples, juiced
1 teaspoon lacuma powder *(see page 16)*
2 teaspoons spirulina powder *(see page 18)*

SERVES 2

Put the blackberries, pears, plums, apple juice, lacuma and spirulina powders in a blender and blend until smooth – simple!

apricots The dried variety, rather than fresh, are a useful source of energy. They may be slightly higher in sugar and calories than fresh, but they are a concentrated source of minerals such as iron and potassium and are richer in fibre, which keeps you full for longer. Sulphur, often used as a preservative in dried apricots, is best avoided, especially by those who suffer from asthma.

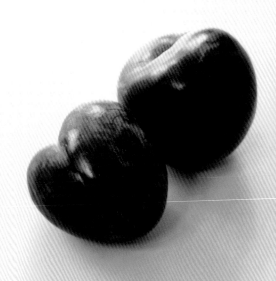

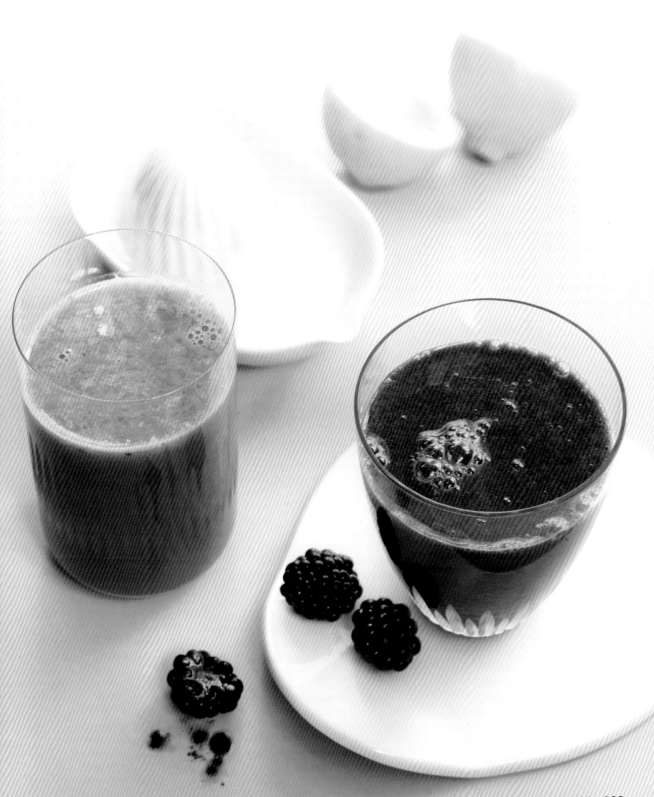

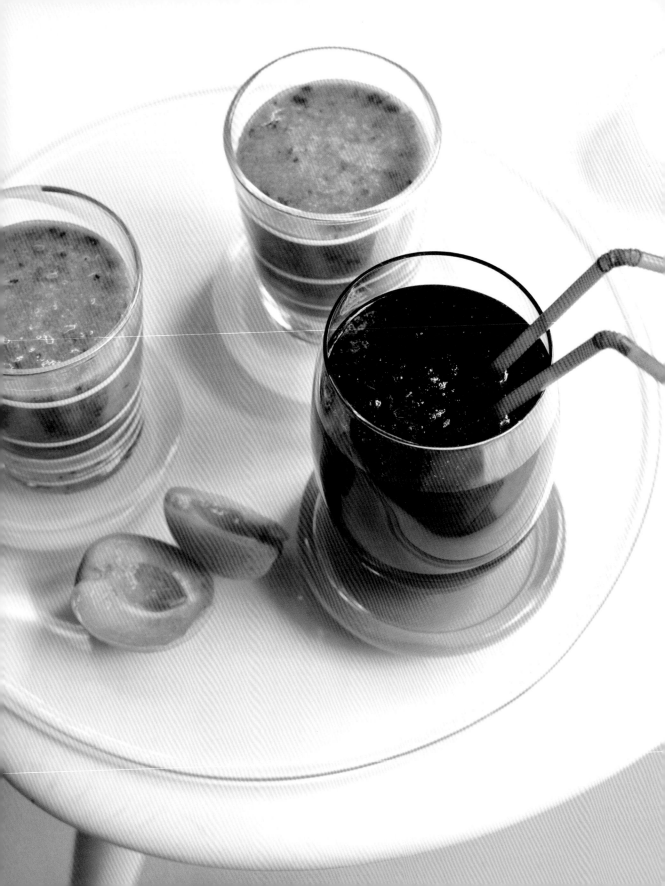

Breakfast to go

Filling, sustaining and a good source of fibre, this drink makes a great start to the day and will provide you with plenty of energy for the morning ahead. Açaí berries have fat-burning properties, reputedly speeding up digestion, reducing cravings and boosting the metabolism.

10 dried ready-to-eat pitted prunes
4 ripe apricots, halved and pitted
juice of 1 red grapefruit
250 ml/1 cup coconut water
juice of ½ lime
2 teaspoons açaí berry powder (*see page 14*)

SERVES 2

Soak the prunes in 50 ml/3½ tablespoons warm water for 30 minutes until softened. Put the prunes and their soaking water, apricots, grapefruit, coconut water, lime juice and açaí berry powder in a blender and blend until smooth.

Coconut quencher

Dehydration can lead to weight gain as our bodies try to retain water and it also contributes to fatigue and brain fog. Additionally, the body can mistake thirst for hunger, increasing the temptation to snack. Coconut water is excellent for rehydrating the body, especially after exercise. I don't peel the pears here as the skin adds valuable nutrients and fibre, but do peel them if the skin is particularly tough.

2 ripe pears, quartered, cored and sliced
2.5-cm/1-inch piece fresh root ginger, peeled
   and finely grated
1 medium beetroot/beet, peeled and grated
350 ml/1½ cups coconut water
1 tablespoon lemon juice
1 teaspoon açaí berry powder (*see page 14*)
1 teaspoon camu camu powder (*see page 15*)

SERVES 2

Put the pears, ginger, beetroot/beet, coconut water, lemon juice, açaí berry powder and camu camu in a blender and blend until smooth.

Cabbage love

If you're not a big fan of green leafy vegetables, the rich texture and tropical flavour of the mango and banana are a real boon. This makes a nutritious and sustaining, get-up-and-go start to the day when energy-levels are low.

2 small handfuls of kale, tough stems discarded, shredded

1 medium mango, peeled, pitted and sliced

1 medium banana, peeled and sliced

2 tablespoons sunflower seeds

1–2 teaspoons spirulina powder (see page 18)

SERVES 2

Put the kale, mango, banana, sunflower seeds and spirulina in a blender with 400 ml/1⅔ cups pure or filtered water, then blend until smooth.

Watermelon heaven

Refreshing, juicy and vibrant, watermelon as its name suggests has a high water content – about 90 per cent – so is especially low in calories. It's also brimming with vitamin C and beta carotene.

1 white tea bag

3 handfuls of cubed, deseeded watermelon

2 handfuls of strawberries, hulled

juice of 1 lime

1 tablespoon ground flaxseeds (see page xx)

½ teaspoon ground ginger

1 tablespoon finely chopped fresh mint

ice cubes, to serve (optional)

SERVES 2

Put the white tea bag in a mug of 200 ml/ generous ¾ cup just-boiled water and allow to infuse for 5 minutes, then remove the tea bag and allow to cool. Just before serving, put the watermelon, strawberries, white tea, lime juice, ground flaxseeds and ground ginger in a blender, then blend until smooth. Stir in the mint and serve on ice.

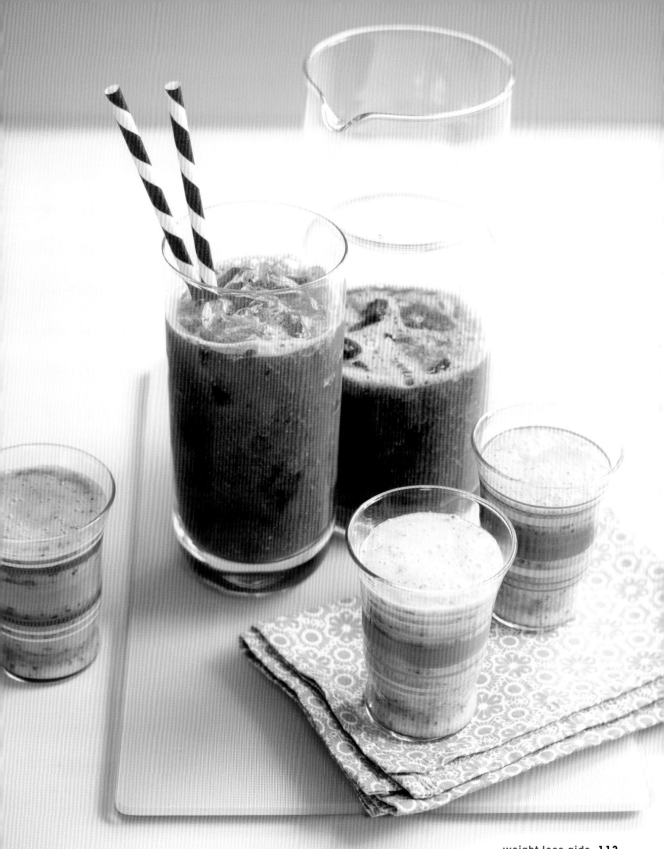

Sweet dreams

The lacuma powder gives a natural sweetness to this smoothie, without the need for adding extra sugar. This recipe can also be adapted to make a delicious fruity yogurt ice, just halve the quantity of nut milk and freeze in a lidded container.

2 handfuls of fresh or frozen
    raspberries
2 handfuls of fresh or frozen
    blueberries
200 ml/generous ¾ cup low-fat
    natural bio yogurt
300 ml/1¼ cups almond milk
    (see page 22)
1 teaspoon vanilla
    extract
1 heaped teaspoon
    lacuma powder
    (see page 16)
2 teaspoons açaí berry powder
    (see page 14)
½ teaspoon chia seeds
    (see page 15) (optional)

SERVES 2

Put the raspberries, blueberries, yogurt, almond milk, vanilla, lacuma and açaí berry powder in a blender and blend until smooth. Serve sprinkled with chia seeds, if you like.

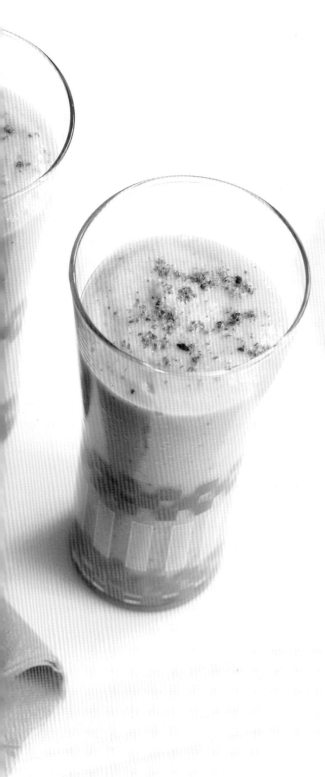

Breakfast in a glass

Providing a beneficial combination of complex carbohydrates, protein, fibre and essential fatty acids, this makes a sustaining, filling breakfast smoothie. Pears with their sweet, almost creamy texture are surprisingly low in calories, which makes them great value when you are craving something sweet, but are keeping an eye on calories.

2 small bananas, peeled and frozen
2 ripe pears, peeled, cored and chopped
200 ml/generous ¾ cup coconut drinking milk
1 tablespoon soya powder or other protein powder
  (see page 18)
seeds from 4 cardamom pods, ground
1 teaspoon ground flaxseeds (see page 16)

SERVES 2

Put the bananas, pears, coconut drinking milk, soya protein, cardamom seeds and half the flaxseeds in a blender and blend until smooth. Serve sprinkled with the remaining flaxseeds.

> **pears** may be low in calories due to their high water content but they provide a wealth of nutrients from vitamins C and K to potassium and manganese. In naturopathic medicine, they are often used as a laxative and diuretic and they are also the most hypoallergenic of fruits, which is useful if you are prone to allergies or intolerances.

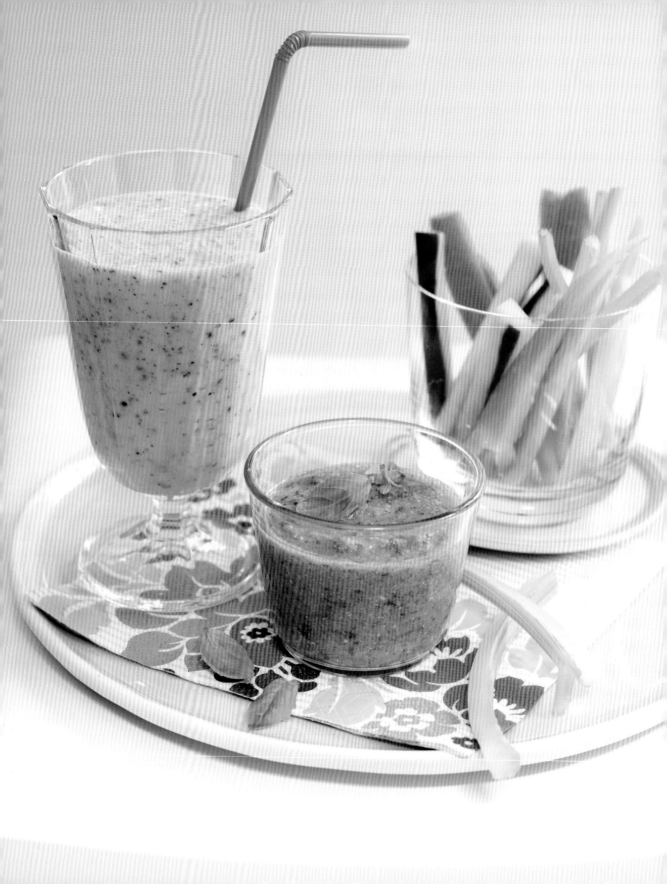

Tropical treat

This makes a great low-fat dessert-cum-smoothie when you're in need of a special low-calorie treat – and it's nutritious.

200 ml/generous ¾ cup low-fat plain bio yogurt
2 passion fruit, halved and fruit scooped out
½ medium mango, peeled, pitted and sliced
200 ml/generous ¾ cup coconut water
½ teaspoon ground ginger
1 tablespoon ground flaxseeds (*see page 16*)
2 teaspoons maca powder (*see page 16*)

SERVES 2

Transfer the yogurt to a freezer-proof container and freeze overnight. Put the frozen yogurt, passion fruit, mango, coconut water, ground ginger, flaxseeds and maca powder in a blender and blend until smooth.

mango This luscious, fragrant fruit tastes indulgent but has a relatively low glycaemic index so will not cause a major spike in blood sugar levels. Like papaya, it contains enzymes that break down protein and aid digestion, helping with uncomfortable bloating. It is also reputed to help cleanse the blood.

Skinny dip

This smoothie-cum-dip makes a quick, calorie-conscious breakfast, lunch or snack. You could leave out, or reduce, the quantity of added water if you want to make a thicker dip, which is perfect for dunking vegetable sticks into.

125 g/generous ½ cup low-fat cottage cheese
1 celery stick, sliced
1 small red (bell) pepper, deseeded and chopped
2 vine-ripened tomatoes, deseeded and sliced
1 handful of basil leaves, plus extra to serve
1 medium red chilli/chile, deseeded and sliced
2 spring onions/scallions, sliced
1 teaspoon ground flaxseeds (*see page 16*)
freshly ground black pepper

SERVES 2

Put the cottage cheese, celery, red (bell) pepper, tomatoes, basil, chilli/chile, spring onions/scallions and ground flaxseed into a blender and blend until almost smooth. Serve topped with extra chopped basil leaves and season with pepper.

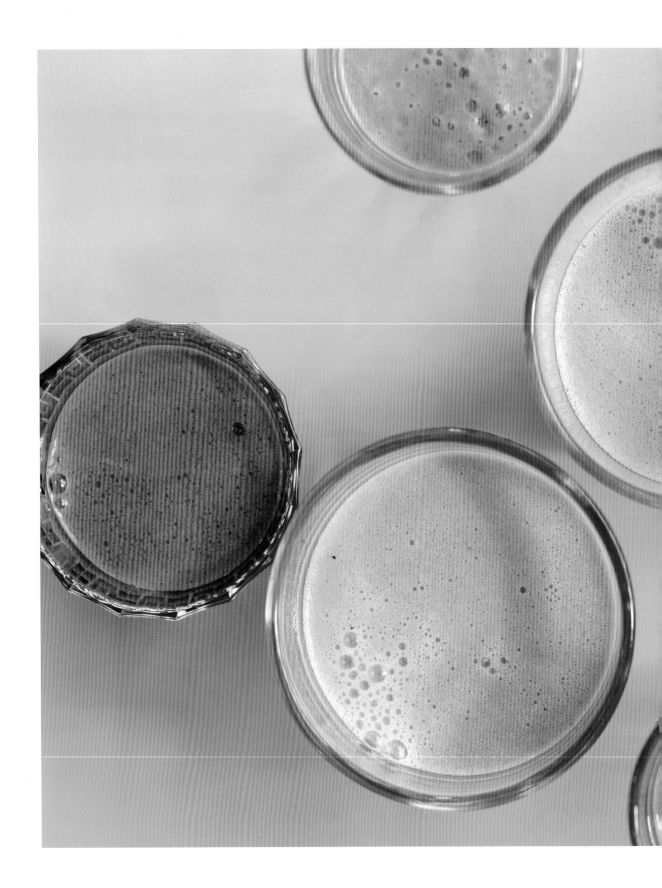

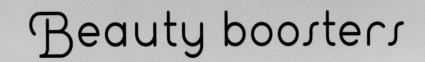

Beauty boosters

Breakfast booster

Hair, skin and nails will all benefit from this vibrant magenta and slightly creamy juice. Vitamin C is important in maintaining collagen levels in the body, which depletes with age leading to wrinkles and poor skin tone. Make sure the fruit is at the peak of ripeness for the best flavour and look for unsweetened coconut water.

1 large pomegranate, quartered and seeds removed
1 large mango, peeled, pitted and sliced
1 large handful of pitted fresh or frozen cherries
300 ml/1¼ cups coconut water
2 teaspoons açaí berry powder (see page 14)
1 teaspoon camu camu powder (see page 15)

SERVES 2

Juice the pomegranate, mango and cherries. Stir in the coconut water, açaí and camu camu powders.

coconut water is the liquid found inside a young, green coconut and is naturally slightly sweet. It is rich in potassium, which enhances the body's ability to hydrate and makes it a useful drink after exercise or indeed if you have a hangover.

Rejuvenator

Bring a glow to your cheeks with one of nature's most effective anti-ageing nutrients. Pink grapefruit and strawberries are packed with vitamin C and this pretty pink juice gets an extra boost from the antioxidant and vitamin C-rich super-fruit, baobab.

1 pink grapefruit
2 large handfuls of strawberries
2 medium pears, cored and sliced
1 teaspoon lemon juice
about 1 teaspoon probiotic powder (see page 18)
   (check recommended dosage on the bottle)
1 teaspoon baobab powder (see page 14)
flaxseeds, for sprinkling

SERVES 2

Juice the grapefruit, strawberries and pears then stir in the lemon juice, probiotic and baobab powders until well combined. Sprinkle the flaxseeds over before serving and feel rejuvenated!

probiotic powders provide 'friendly' bacteria such as *lactobacillus acidophilus* and *bifidus* to stimulate sluggish or poor digestion and improve the absorption of nutrients. A healthy gut is important in curbing 'bad' bacteria and conditions related to yeast overgrowth, such as candida and if you are healthy on the inside you're more likely to look healthy on the outside.

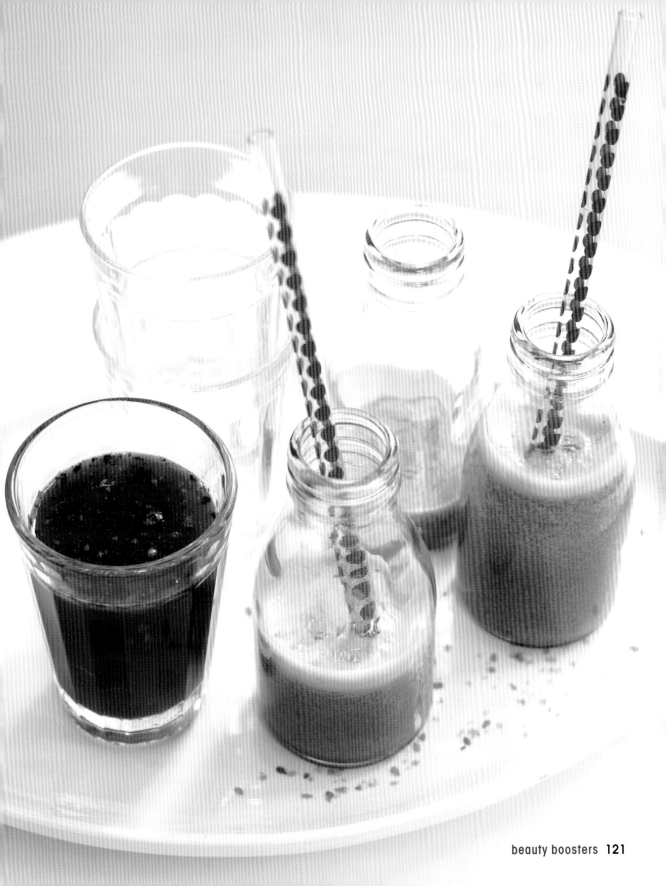

Coco-loco

Making juices and smoothies with infused spices such as cloves, cinnamon and ginger takes a little extra time, but you will be rewarded with a wonderful depth of flavour.

300 ml/1¼ cups coconut drinking milk

1 stick lemongrass, bruised

2 cloves

1 stick cinnamon

1-cm/³⁄₈-inch piece fresh root ginger, unpeeled
   and sliced

½ large pineapple, peeled, cored and
   cut into long wedges

2 teaspoons lacuma powder (*see page 16*)

½ teaspoon toasted unsweetened desiccated
   coconut, for sprinkling

SERVES 2

Pour the coconut milk into a pan and add the lemongrass, cloves, cinnamon and ginger. Heat over a medium-low heat until just warm then turn off the heat, cover with a lid and leave to infuse for 1 hour (or overnight if making the next morning). Strain and discard the lemongrass, cloves, cinnamon and ginger. Juice the pineapple and stir in the infused milk and the lacuma. Pour into glasses and sprinkle with the coconut.

spices have been valued for their medicinal properties for many thousands of years, particularly for their digestive, antibacterial, antiseptic and antiviral qualities. They taste great, too…

In the pink

Your hair, skin and nails will love this blended juice, which is bursting with vitamins A and C, fibre, antioxidants and phytonutrients. A lack of these nutrients, particularly vitamin A, can result in a dry scalp and possibly lead to hair loss.

100 ml/⅓ cup coconut water

3 large handfuls of chopped, deseeded watermelon

2 large handfuls of strawberries, hulled

1 large carrot, peeled and grated

½ teaspoon flaxseed oil

1–2 teaspoons spirulina powder (*see page 18*)

SERVES 2

Put the coconut water in a blender with the watermelon, strawberries, carrot, flaxseed oil and spirulina and blend until smooth.

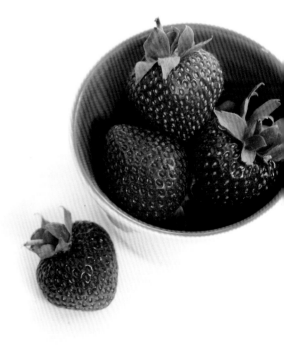

Hair gloss

One of the few fruits to contain vitamin E, blackberries are also a good source of vitamin C, a beneficial combination that helps to protect the skin against UV damage from the sun. MSM, a natural form of sulphur found in leafy green vegetables and sold as a supplement, helps with eczema, acne, psoriasis and dandruff and its effectiveness is enhanced by taking vitamin C and camu camu at the same time.

1 small cantaloupe melon, deseeded, sliced into
   long wedges and skin removed
2 handfuls of blackberries
1 large orange, peeled and divided
   into segments
2 teaspoons chopped mint leaves
½ –1 teaspoon MSM powder (see page 17)
1 teaspoon camu camu powder (see page 15)

SERVES 2

Juice the melon, blackberries and orange, then stir in the mint, MSM and camu camu powders.

Green goddess

The watercress gives a spicy kick to this vibrant green juice, which is a winning combination created to help tone and beautify the skin as well as give strong, healthy hair and nails.

6 green apples, peeled, cored and cut into wedges
4 handfuls of watercress, large stalks removed
4 handfuls of flat-leaf parsley, stalks removed
1 small handful of alfalfa sprouts (see page 21)
juice of 1 small lemon
1–2 teaspoons spirulina (see page 18)

SERVES 2

Juice the apples. Using a stick blender, blend together the watercress, parsley, alfalfa sprouts and lemon juice, then add to the apple juice and stir in the spirulina.

watercress With impressive levels of beta carotene, iron, vitamin C, B vitamins and phytochemicals, watercress gives us healthy skin, hair, nails, bones and teeth.

melon The orange-fleshed cantaloupe melon is rich in beta carotene and vitamin C and is also a good source of silicon, a trace mineral important for maintaining healthy skin.

cabbage Leafy greens are packed with nutrients, particularly phytochemicals, which are a collection of beneficial compounds found in fresh vegetables. Cabbage is particularly potent juiced or eaten raw and has antibacterial and antiviral properties.

Skin detox

If your juicer struggles with leafy greens, it's a good idea to alternate adding the greens with the grapes, to help it on its way. Spinach and cabbage are a surprising source of omega-3 fats, which help to keep skin healthy and plump.

2 handfuls of seedless white grapes
4 handfuls of spinach leaves
2 pears, peeled, cored and cut into long wedges
4 handfuls of sweetheart cabbage, shredded
2 teaspoons lemon juice
2 teaspoons powdered greens (*see page 17*)

SERVES 2

Juice the grapes, spinach, pears and cabbage. Stir in the lemon juice and powdered greens.

Skin brightener

This deliciously fruity, pink juice is rejuvenating and nutritious. Goji berries, despite their diminutive size, are a small powerhouse of nutrients and are particularly good for the health of the eyes.

4 tablespoons goji berries
3 handfuls of strawberries, hulled
½ medium pineapple, peeled, cored and cut into chunks
1–2 teaspoons camu camu powder (*see page 15*)
100 ml/⅓ cup sparkling mineral water

SERVES 2

Soak the goji berries in 4 tablespoons pure or filtered water for 15 minutes until softened, then tip them and the soaking water into a blender with the strawberries, pineapple and camu camu and blend until smooth. Stir in the sparkling water and serve.

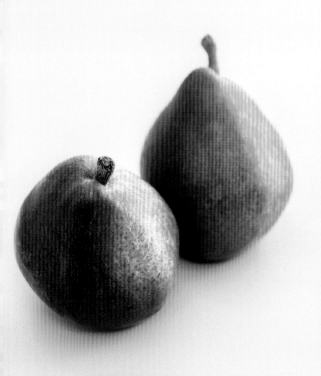

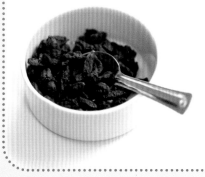

goji berries Great for boosting the immune system, goji berries contain, weight for weight, more vitamin C than oranges, more iron than steak and more beta carotene than carrots – impressive!

Purple days

Purple corn is a Peruvian superfood brimming with health benefits, and has an even higher antioxidant content than blueberries. It has been shown to boost collagen formation and protect capillaries so is especially beneficial for the skin.

2 handfuls of blueberries
2 handfuls of fresh or frozen blackberries
2 handfuls of strawberries, hulled
1 teaspoon bilberry powder (*see page 18*)
2 teaspoons açaí berry powder (*see page 14*)
1 teaspoon lacuma powder (*see page 16*)
1–2 teaspoons purple corn powder (*see page 17*)

SERVES 2

Put the blueberries, blackberries, strawberries, bilberry powder, açaí berry powder, lacuma and purple corn powder into a blender and blend until smooth – you can pass it through a sieve to remove the seeds if you wish. If preferred, add pure or filtered water if too thick. It can also be served as a fruit coulis, stirred into plain bio yogurt or with added nuts, seeds, grains and a spoonful of manuka honey for breakfast.

Protein smoothie

Protein is essential for the repair and maintenance of every cell in the body and that includes the skin, hair and nails. This protein-boosting smoothie makes an energising start to the day and while you could opt for soya or pea protein instead, hemp protein powder is additionally a good source of minerals and omega-3 fats.

2 medium bananas, peeled
1 handful of blanched almonds
1 carrot, peeled and coarsely grated
2 pears, peeled, cored and chopped
½ teaspoon ground cinnamon
2 teaspoons chopped fresh root ginger
2 teaspoons hemp protein powder (*see page 18*)

SERVES 2

Wrap the bananas in plastic wrap and freeze overnight. Soak the almonds in 100 ml/⅓ cup pure or filtered water overnight. The next day, remove the bananas from the freezer, unwrap and allow to soften for a few minutes. Chop the bananas and put in a blender with the almonds and soaking water, an extra 350 ml/1½ cups pure or filtered water, carrot, pears, cinnamon, ginger and hemp protein powder. Blend until smooth.

blackberries In natural medicine, blackberries are used to cleanse the blood, treat menstrual problems and stomach complaints and as a tonic. Rich in bioflavonoids, blackberries are also one of the best low-fat sources of vitamin E.

Skin freshener

Barleygrass is known to improve the condition of the skin and is helped here by the hydrating effect of the cucumber and coconut water. This makes a refreshing, cooling, summery drink, especially if served on ice.

4 kiwi fruits, peeled and halved

1 small cucumber, deseeded and chopped

275 ml/1 cup plus 1 tablespoon coconut water

juice of ½ lime

1 small handful of mint leaves

2 tablespoons flaked quinoa

1–2 teaspoons barleygrass powder (*see page 14*)

1.5-cm/⅝-inch piece fresh root ginger, peeled
and finely grated

SERVES 2

Put the kiwi, cucumber, coconut water, lime juice, mint, quinoa and barleygrass into a blender. Squeeze the ginger through a muslin/cheesecloth bag or your fingers to extract the juice and add to the blender. Blend until smooth.

quinoa Hailed a 'supergrain', quinoa is different from other grains in that it's a complete protein. It is also an excellent source of iron, calcium, potassium, B vitamins, magnesium and zinc.

Wrinkle killer

You can keep the skin on the apples if you like as it adds valuable fibre and nutrients and is almost undetectable when blended. Skin problems are said to benefit from eating apples on a regular basis, which is no doubt due to their ability to purify the blood, while pears and cherries have also been praised for giving a clear complexion and glossy hair.

2 pears, peeled, cored and chopped

2 apples, quartered, cored and chopped

2 handfuls of frozen pitted dark cherries

1–2 teaspoons wheatgrass powder (*see page 18*)

2 teaspoons cranberry powder (*see page 18*)

SERVES 2

Put the pears, apples, cherries, wheatgrass powder and cranberry powder in a blender with 250 ml/1 cup pure or filtered water and blend until smooth.

apples This humble fruit gives us an immense list of health benefits from reducing tooth decay by lowing levels of bacteria in the mouth to cutting levels of harmful LDL cholesterol and curbing the risk of cancer of the colon, liver and breast.

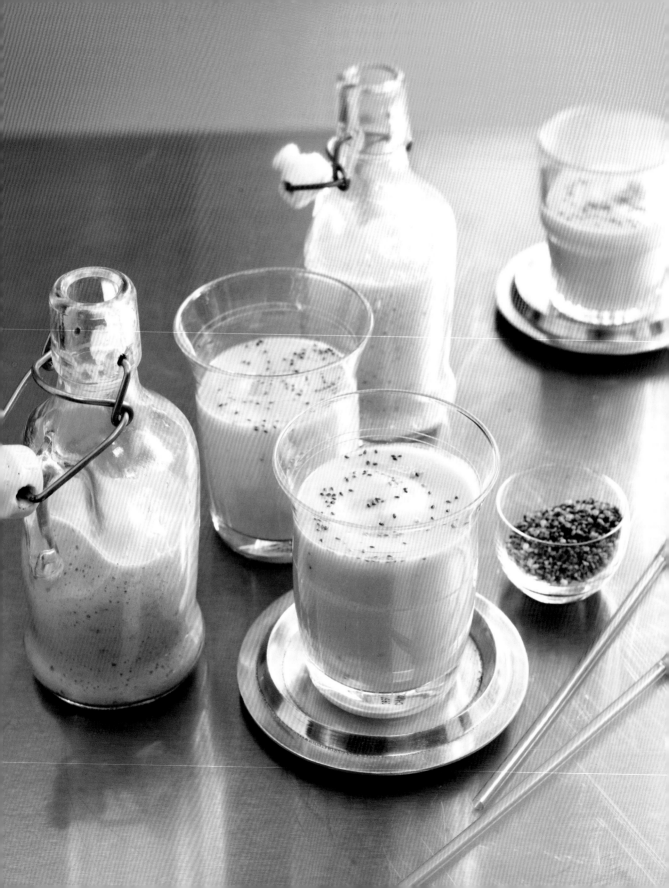

Apricot smoother

A creamy, filling smoothie that doubles-up as a delicious dessert if you're looking for something sweet and nutritious. You could freeze the bananas first, then use from frozen to make a sort of healthy ice cream – do peel them first.

6 unsulphured dried apricots
2 medium bananas, peeled and broken into pieces
150 ml/^{2}/$_3$ cup plain bio yogurt
½ teaspoon vanilla extract
100 ml/^{1}/$_3$ cup coconut drinking milk
2 teaspoons maca powder (*see page 16*)
bee pollen (*see page 15*), for sprinkling

SERVES 2

Soak the apricots in 100 ml/^{1}/$_3$ cup of pure or filtered water for 30 minutes (or overnight if making the smoothie the next day). Put the apricots, bananas, yogurt, vanilla extract, coconut drinking milk and maca powder in a blender and blend until smooth.
Sprinkle with bee pollen before serving.

Green and plenty

Avocado gives a delicious creaminess to this smoothie and combines surprisingly well with the fresh mango and aromatic lime, but make sure it is nice and ripe for the best results.

1 small mango, peeled, pitted and cut into chunks
1 medium avocado, peeled, pitted and sliced
300 ml/1¼ cups almond milk (*see page 22*)
juice of 1 large lime
seeds from 3 cardamom pods, ground
¼ teaspoon chia seeds (*see page 15*), for sprinkling

SERVES 2

Put the mango, avocado, almond milk and lime juice in a blender and blend until smooth. Stir in the ground cardamom seeds and serve sprinkled with chia seeds.

avocados are great for improving the condition of the skin, hair and nails with their beneficial amounts of vitamins C and E as well as iron, potassium and manganese. They also provide lutein, a carotenoid that works as an antioxidant to help protect against eye disease. Some people avoid the avocados due to their relatively high fat content, but it is the heart-friendly monounsaturated type and good for your skin, too.

Skin smooth-ie

Not only do avocados lend a lovely creaminess to smoothies, they are known for their ability to improve the condition of the skin and hair – a double whammy!

1 small avocado, halved, pitted, peeled and sliced
2 pears, cored and chopped (peeled, if liked)
350 ml/1½ cups almond milk (*see page 22*)
1 heaped teaspoon manuka honey (*see page 16*)
1 teaspoon ground cinnamon
probiotic powder (*see page 18*)
  (*check the recommended dosage on the bottle*)
1 tablespoon lemon juice

SERVES 2

Put the avocado, pears, almond milk, honey, cinnamon, probiotic powder and lemon juice in a blender and blend until smooth.

Rosy cheeks smoothie

I prefer to use frozen raspberries, rather than buy fresh fruit when it's not in season. In fact, it's a good idea to keep a ready supply of frozen fruit for smoothies or juices. There's no need to defrost the fruit, just throw a handful into the blender straight from the freezer.

2 large handfuls of fresh or frozen raspberries
2 pears, peeled, cored and chopped
150 ml/⅔ cup fresh apple juice (not from
  concentrate) or 2 small apples, juiced
125 ml/½ cup plain bio yogurt
1 tablespoon soya protein (*see page 18*)
2 teaspoons camu camu powder (*see page 15*)
¼ teaspoon freshly grated nutmeg, plus extra to serve

SERVES 2

Put the raspberries, pears, apple juice, yogurt, soya protein, camu camu powder and grated nutmeg in a blender and blend until smooth and creamy. Served sprinkled with a little extra nutmeg.

peaches Much of a peach's vitamin C content lies within or just below the skin so it makes sense to eat the fruit unpeeled. Our own skin benefits from the high levels of this vitamin as well as beta carotene and a wide range of minerals.

Smooth as a peach

Aromatic with spices, this tropical-tasting smoothie is pure indulgence in a glass. Make sure the peaches are in the peak of ripeness for the best flavour – I don't bother removing the skin as many of the fruit's nutrients lie just under the skin and life is too short!

2 tablespoons goji berries

3 large ripe peaches, halved, pitted and chopped

250 ml/1 cup coconut drinking milk

300 ml/1¼ cups plain bio yogurt

1 teaspoon orange flower water, or to taste

seeds from 3 cardamom pods, crushed

½ teaspoon freshly grated nutmeg

1 heaped tablespoon unsalted shelled pistachio nuts,
    plus extra to serve

1 teaspoon camu camu powder (*see page 15*)

1 teaspoon baobab powder (*see page 14*)

5 ice cubes

SERVES 2

Soak the goji berries in 2 tablespoons pure or filtered water for 15 minutes until softened. Put the goji and their soaking water in a blender with the peaches, coconut drinking milk, yogurt, orange flower water, cardamom seeds, nutmeg, pistachios, camu camu, baobab powder and ice, then blend until smooth. Serve sprinkled with chopped pistachios.

Strawberry and cinnamon lassi

This smoothie is luxuriously creamy with just a hint of rose. If your blender struggles with ice cubes, you can crush them in a bag using the end of a rolling pin, then add to the blender with the rest of the ingredients.

300 ml/1¼ cups plain bio yogurt

3 handfuls of strawberries, hulled

1 teaspoon rose flower water, or to taste

1 tablespoon ground flaxseeds (*see page 16*)

1 teaspoon ground cinnamon

2 teaspoons manuka honey (*see page 16*)

probiotic powder (*see page 18*)
    (*check the recommended dosage on the bottle*)

8 ice cubes

bee pollen, for sprinkling (*see page 15*)

SERVES 2

Put the yogurt, strawberries, rose flower water, ground flaxseeds, cinnamon, honey, probiotic powder and ice cubes in a blender and blend until smooth and creamy. Serve sprinkled with bee pollen.

manuka honey Studies on manuka honey have revealed its potent antiviral, antibacterial, anti-inflammatory, antimicrobial, antiseptic and antifungal properties, which are over and above that of regular honey. Look for an UMF (Unique Manuka Factor) of at least 10+ on the label for the most active health properties.

Turn back the clock

MSM, a natural form of sulphur, is often referred to as the 'beauty mineral'. While the nutrient is found in green leafy vegetables, many of us are deficient in MSM, so it may be wise to consider a supplement to boost levels. It helps with the formation of collagen, elastin, cartilage and keratin, benefitting the skin, nails and hair.

4 tablespoons goji berries
250 ml/1 cup coconut water
3 passion fruits, halved and fruit scooped out
2 large bananas, peeled and sliced
½–1 teaspoon MSM powder (*see page 17*)
1–2 teaspoons maca (*see page 16*)

SERVES 2

Soak the goji berries in 100 ml/⅓ cup pure or filtered water for 15 minutes until softened then tip into a blender with the coconut water, passion fruits, bananas, MSM powder and maca then blend until smooth – there will be small flecks from the passion fruit seeds.

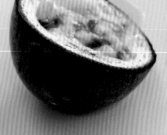

passion fruit This fruit is rich in vitamin C, beta carotene and other antioxidants, which are all crucial for maintaining healthy skin, good vision and preventing premature ageing. A single fruit will supply all the vitamin C you need for one day!

Black forest smoothie

Chocolate, cherries and raspberries taste great together and, as an added bonus, are a healthy mix of antioxidants, fibre, vitamins and minerals. The skin will benefit from their ability to cleanse and revive.

3 good handfuls of frozen pitted dark cherries
1 good handful of raspberries
1 large handful of baby spinach leaves
400 ml/1⅔ cups plain bio yogurt
½ teaspoon ground cinnamon
1 teaspoon raw cacao powder (*see page 15*)
1 teaspoon vanilla extract
1 tablespoon toasted oats, sprinkled on top

SERVES 2

Put the cherries, raspberries, spinach, yogurt, cinnamon, cacao powder and vanilla into a blender and blend until smooth. Serve sprinkled with the toasted oats.

oats To keep your digestive system healthy, it pays to eat oats on a regular basis. Their fibre content will also help to reduce levels of harmful LDL cholesterol, while increasing beneficial HDL cholesterol.

Index

Suppliers

UK SOURCES

BLUE HERBS
020 3488 3830
sales@blueherbs.co.uk
www.blueherbs.co.uk
A range of fine, first class products, each one designed to enhance health, wellbeing and quality of life.

DETOX TRADING
01803 762368
orders@detoxtrading.co.uk
www.detoxtrading.co.uk
Supply high quality, organic (UK Soil Association Certified) superfoods.

FUNKY RAW
shop@funkyraw.com
www.funkyraw.com
Online raw food shop.

JOHN LEWIS
www.johnlewis.com/juicers
All kinds of equipment for juicing and blending.

JUICE MASTER
www.juicemaster.com
One-stop shop for all your juicing needs.

RAW GAIA
01273 311476
www.rawgaia.com
The world's premier all organic, raw and vegan skin care company.

SUPERFOOD DIRECT
01273 771127
www.thesuperfooddirect.com
Supplier of organic superfoods.

THE SUPERFOOD COMPANY
0118 947 1387
www.thesuperfoodco.co.uk
Suppliers of superfoods, powders, capsules and teas along with a wide range of branded supplements and alternative natural health products and remedies.

UK JUICERS
www.ukjuicers.com
Impressive range of juicers and blenders for all budgets.

WHOLEFOODS
www.wholefoodsmarket.com
Suppliers of organic fresh foods and superfoods.

US SOURCES

CRATE & BARREL
www.crateandbarrel.com
Stylish juicing equipment, tableware and more.

EREWHON
www.erewhonmarket.com
Healthy, pure, nutrient-rich foods.

THE FRESH MARKET
www.thefreshmarket.com
Over 100 stores supplying fresh, delicious products.

SPOONS N SPICE
www.spoonsnspice.com
Quality kitchenware. Ship across the United States.

SUNFOOD
www.sunfood.com
Raw organic non-GMO superfoods.

SUR LA TABLE
www.surlatable.com
Stylish, extensive range of juicing equipment.

TRADER JOE'S
www.traderjoes.com
Speciality grocery stores.

WEGMANS
www.wegmans.com
High-quality fresh produce and superfoods.

WHOLEFOODS
www.wholefoodsmarket.com
Suppliers of organic fresh foods and superfoods.

WILLIAMS-SONOMA
www.williams-sonoma.com
A wealth of juicing equipment from smoothie makers to wheatgrass juicers.

Acknowledgments

Thank you to Nick Ledger at UK Juicers for supplying the Champion juicer. This centrifugal juicer is a real beast of a machine and efficiently handled most fruit and vegetables at a press of a button. Check out the UK Juicers' website as they supply an impressive range of juicers and blenders for all budgets.

www.ukjuicers.com

I would also like to thank Magimix for supplying the Le Blender. Along with making easy work of smoothies and blended drinks, it's a great everyday blender for making soups and frozen desserts and comes with a mill attachment for grinding spices and nuts, and making breadcrumbs, sauces and dips.

www.magimix.com

I have to acknowledge Tree Harvest, who supply a wide range of superfoods as well as a whole host of wonderful herbs, dried fruit, berries, seeds, nuts, fruit and vegetable powders, oils... and the list goes on. A truly ethical company and always a pleasure to deal with, their contact details are below. (They don't have a website but you can download their catalogue.)

enquiries@tree-harvest.com

My heartfelt thanks go to Julia Charles, editorial director at Ryland, Peters & Small for giving me the opportunity to write this book and for her continued support over the years. I would also like show my appreciation to Miriam Catley, who calmly and efficiently worked on the text; designers Toni Kay (it's been a long time) and Megan Smith; photographer Kate Whitaker, with her truly inspiring and inventive shots; and food stylist Lucy McKelvie. A big thank you also goes to Anneli Fleming-Brown who helped me with testing and came up with many inspired suggestions.